T IS FOR TRANSFORMATION

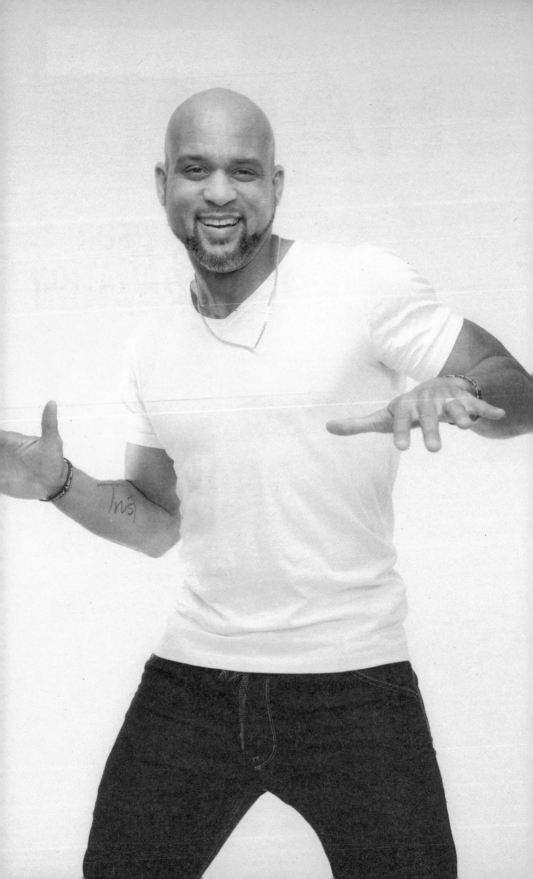

Advance Praise for
T Is for Transformation

"*T Is for Transformation* is so much more than just a personal memoir. I finished the book feeling like a better version of me. I've been lucky enough to have Shaun T as a personal mentor and friend for years, so it was no surprise to FEEL his motivation exploding out the pages of his book."

—Bob Ruff,
host of the Truth & Justice *podcast*

"Shaun has helped millions of people transform their bodies and change their lives. And he's the most genuine, down-to-earth dude you'll ever meet. I can't recommend his book enough to people who want to take control of their lives and maximize what they've got."

—BJ Gaddour,
Men's Health *fitness director*

"Shaun T is the most caring person in this world, and his book will be life changing for those who truly want to dig deep and transform even if they've had a rough go at life so far. You just gotta Trust and Believe in Shaun T and he will show you the way."

—Drew Manning,
New York Times *bestselling author of* Fit2Fat2Fit

"This book gives you the tools you need to understand that nothing comes easy, but anything is possible. It is NOT a book about Shaun T—it's about *you*. His life story is the conduit through which you can achieve your dreams. Now I have answers to my biggest challenges and so will you."

—Eddie Nestor,
host of BBC Radio London's Drivetime with Eddie Nestor

"Not only has Shaun inspired millions of people to transform their bodies, his incredible personal transformation in this book will no doubt help millions more transform their souls and hearts, as well."

—*Harley Pasternak,*
celebrity trainer and New York Times *bestselling author of* The Body Reset Diet

"*T Is for Transformation* is a testament to the fact that within every obstacle there is opportunity. Shaun T is a life changer—I dare you to read this book and not want to take on the world."

—Andrea Boehlke, *Survivor* contestant and host of *PEOPLE Now*

"Shaun T is in a class by himself and knows the struggles we all face day-to-day. Having been fortunate enough to work with him on set, this book *T Is for Transformation* encompasses all the magic and positivity he exudes in person, while giving the mental tools we all need to succeed."

—Albert Bianchini, executive producer, Milojo Productions

"As someone who knows Shaun T well, I still found myself deep into this book finding out even more about him than I knew before and being motivated and inspired in new ways. I finished this book feeling inspired to take action, ready to tackle my life, and motivated to truly trust and believe in who I am."

—*Danielle Natoni,*
creator of Fit & Funky *and* Beachbody LIVE Master Trainer

"To see Shaun fight his way out of the darkest of places not only inspires me to be braver, it shows me that no matter what life has in store for us, we can all have a Secret Backpack and can unleash our superpowers whenever we are faced with life struggles and challenges."

—*Tania Baron,*
founder of Team Machine *and* Beachbody LIVE Master Trainer

SHAUN T

T IS FOR TRANSFORMATION

UNLEASH THE
7 SUPERPOWERS TO
HELP YOU DIG DEEPER,
FEEL STRONGER &
LIVE YOUR BEST LIFE

Vermilion
LONDON

1 3 5 7 9 10 8 6 4 2

Vermilion, an imprint of Ebury Publishing,
20 Vauxhall Bridge Road,
London SW1V 2SA

Vermilion is part of the Penguin Random House group of companies whose
addresses can be found at global.penguinrandomhouse.com

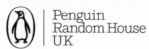
Penguin
Random House
UK

First published in the United Kingdom by Vermilion in 2017
First published in the USA by Rodale 2017

www.penguin.co.uk

A CIP catalogue record for this book is available from the British Library

ISBN 9781785041631

Printed and bound in Great Britain by Clays Ltd, St Ives PLC

Penguin Random House is committed to a sustainable future for our business,
our readers and our planet. This book is made from Forest Stewardship
Council® certified paper.

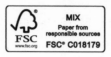

CONTENTS

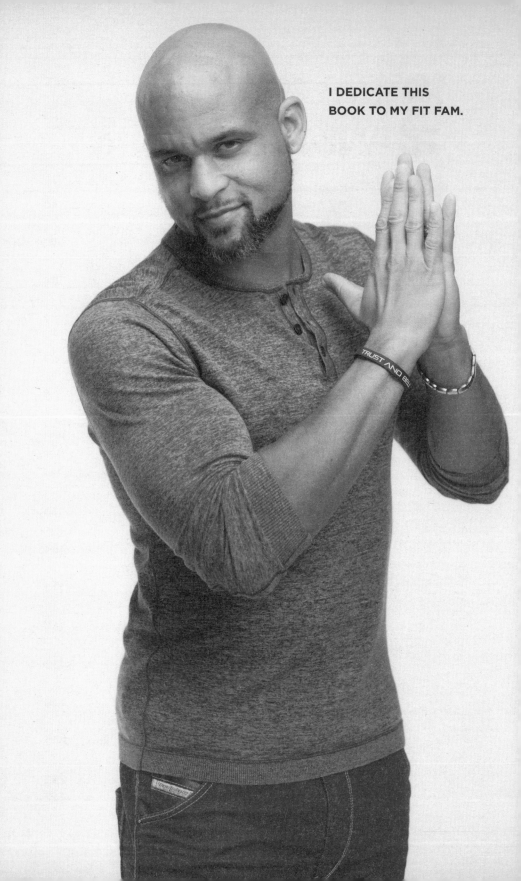

I DEDICATE THIS
BOOK TO MY FIT FAM.

AN INVITATION TO
TRANSFORMATION

Congratulations.

"For what?" you ask. Making it all the way to page 1?

Yes, exactly.

Congratulations for being motivated to start on your personal transformation. And for trying to turn the page on everything that has been holding you back.

That's amazeballs.

But, congratulations as well for being whoever you are right now. People who are willing to take the first step toward life transformation are the strongest people in the world.

The more struggles you've had, the stronger you can be.

IT DOESN'T MATTER IF YOU'RE LOOKING forward to your fifth go-around with *INSANITY.*® Or if you pressed play on one of my workout programs and thought: *Insane is right. I'm not doing that.*

Because the kind of fitness I care most about is *inside you*.

It's in your mind.

It's in your heart.

And both of those are great places to find strength, because you're in charge there. Nobody else can tell you what to do, or who you are, or how strong you can be.

It's all up to you.

Can you screen out the noise in your life to hear what you need to?

Can you push away the people that tell you it can't be done, and decide for yourself what you can achieve?

Can you trust yourself to handle the stress of change? Can you believe in your ability to succeed now, even if you've fallen short before?

TRUST AND BELIEVE.

You can see why I keep on going back to those two words. They're the engines that get me out of bed every day, knowing that I'll be a little farther along toward my goals by bedtime.

You may have to train yourself to trust yourself, and the time to start that training is now. Not that every day will be great. But, even if I have a disappointment or a setback or an injury, I know that trusting and believing will help me understand why I failed, and I formulate a plan to overcome it.

THIS ISN'T A GET-YOUR-SH!T-TOGETHER BOOK.

It's a place where you'll gather life-changing tools and learn to use them.

It won't happen quickly. Nothing worth achieving ever does.

But, I promise you that it's going to *feel so good* as you move forward that nobody will be able to stop you.

So, don't rush the process. Enjoy it.

You have the power to turn your struggles into strength.

It all starts here.

Trust and believe: *You can do this.*

CHAPTER ONE

THE SEVEN SUPERPOWERS

This book isn't about me. It's about you.

I want to share my life story to show you what I've been through and how I handled it, so that you know that I've been there. I want you to believe that the lessons I learned from my challenges can cross over into the life you're living, and they can help you figure out where you want to go from here.

You have frustrations? So do I.

You've fallen short of your goals? Me, too.

You've been disappointed by the people closest to you? Read *on*.

But this isn't only about failures and screw-ups.

It's about that awesome feeling when you lose the first 4 pounds on a weight-loss journey.

Or, when you find a love that surprised you with its intensity.

Or, when your job provides rewards that go way beyond the paycheck.

You see where I'm going?

Shaun T has been there and done all of that—downside, and upside.

Sometimes, it feels like we're on a hamster wheel, running as fast as we can and ending up exhausted but in the same place as we've always been. Listen up: I know about rat racing. Neither of us should go there, and it's time to get off the wheel!

Unless . . . being a rodent is just a step along the way to an amazeballs outcome you couldn't have imagined; I actually played a rodent on stage (see Chapter Five), and that experience taught me a lot. But more on that later.

It's past time to step off that wheel and make *real* progress. I'm not just talking about building a six pack or losing 100 pounds or shutting up your annoying sister-in-law. Here's what I want: for you to identify what's actually important *to you*, to find a way to achieve that, and to make your gains an authentic part of who you are. That kind of growth and progress will last the rest of your life, and nobody can ever take it away.

To help you build your transformation toolbox, I'll be giving you a test that will help you learn more about who you are, plus exercises to help you find pathways from where you are to where you want to be. I'll be asking what you want out of your life, and challenging you to figure out what's holding you back. I'll also suggest strategies and life experiments that can move you forward.

By the end of this book, you will have built interior strength—the only kind that really sticks with you—to fend off failures, answer the haters, and give you the energy to move upward. I'm also going to give you some tools to build your physical strength, because, sometimes, it helps to practice pushing yourself physically in order to get better at doing it mentally.

People always ask me: What is the key is to losing weight—exercise or diet? I always tell them: "Neither. The most important thing is *your mind*, and that's a muscle you can build just like any other."

I'm here to help you build yours, starting with two key truthbombs:

TRUTHBOMB: The only meaningful obstacles are mental ones.

TRUTHBOMB: Nothing looks as good as confidence feels.

Whatever your goal is—losing weight, finding your life's work, meeting The One, tapping into your passions—you're now on the path to achieving them.

The pathway of your life may wander a bit, and that's okay: It can go anywhere you want it to.

Mine has wandered . . . a lot. That's why I'm going to tell my story—the good, the bad, and the ugly—and I'm not going to hold anything back. It's the only way I know how to be.

Parts of my life story are embarrassing for me. But even the most difficult things that have happened to me have made me who I am today. If not for the bad parts, I never would have made it to the best parts. And the best parts are worth looking at, too, because they flow in a direct line from the worst. I'm not complaining about anything. I'm celebrating the good, and acknowledging how it sprang directly from my biggest struggles.

If you bury your painful experiences deep, or hide them in the closet, or deny them completely, you'll never be able to move past them.

I'll never do that again. It hasn't always been that way for me, as you'll see.

But right now, I'm asking: What are *you* hiding from yourself and others? What pain, embarrassment, or difficulty are you holding onto because letting go of it seems too hard? Trust me: I know what that struggle feels like.

If you're holding something back, it's holding you back—from true happiness now, from the better future you dream of. If you don't deal with the most difficult aspects of your life, past or present, you'll keep living them every day you have left.

TRUTHBOMB: You get stronger by unpacking the baggage, not by stuffing it into the closet.

People see me today, smiling on Facebook or leading a workout, and they're thinking, *this is easy for him*. I'm here to tell you, *nothing* was *easy* about getting Shaun T where he is today, and it still ain't easy.

And anyway, *easy* isn't the point.

The pain is.

The work is.

The process is.

And finally, the progress is.

THERE'S NO BETTER PLACE TO STUDY human motivation than a workout studio. I've led thousands of workouts in my life, so I'm super-sensitive to what holds people back, and also what allows them to break through. The people who fail do it in the same old ways—negative self-talk, not showing up, excuse-making—and those who succeed show similar strengths: scheduling workouts, setting goals, recruiting a supportive posse. Just as developing certain muscle groups and cardio endurance can help you get through an *INSANITY* session, developing certain skills can help you move on to a whole new life. And that means helping you to help *yourself*.

Think about that word "core" for a minute. You've heard thousands of exercise coaches talk about the need for core strength. I talk about it a lot, too. But what I really care most about is your personal core—the values that drive your choices, the people you surround yourself with, your attitude toward yourself. The same way strong abs and back muscles support every move you make, a strong personal core can help you move decisively into your future. It's your choice: You'll either suffer with every move, or go strong into the future.

That's why you have to learn:

What's important to you.

Who's important to you.

What's driving you forward.

What's promising to take you to that place you've only dreamed about, but didn't dare expect for yourself.

There are core exercises that can give you a six pack, and there are core exercises that can give you the strength to absorb the gut punches life delivers. I've shaped plenty of abdomens in the last 20 years. Now, I want to empower you to reshape your life by working at what's most important to you. Your core values.

Change has knocked me sideways plenty of times, but then, success is seldom a straight line. You can zig and zag your way to the promised land. In fact, there's no other way to get there.

BAD TIMES ARE LIKE BOOT CAMP. You go through them to build up strength—to reach a better place. Every tough step you take moves you forward, and the tougher they are, the more strength you build and the greater the leap you can make.

I'll help you find the purpose to your pitfalls, as you learn about my hard times, too. Like I say in my workouts: Use your own body to build your body. It's the same with every difficult thing you've done and experienced. Use your life—whatever it brings—to build your life. When strength comes from within, nobody can take it from you.

Not the relative who molested you.

Not the spouse who beat you.

Not the boss who harassed you.

Not the mean kids who bullied you.

Not the people who counted you out, told you that you didn't matter, brushed you aside.

When you build the strength to move past those people, or climb over an obstacle, you have a new superpower nobody can take from you. I've been building new superpowers since I was a little kid, and now I use them everywhere I go. When another big challenge or problem comes up, I deploy what I need to overcome it or make it disappear.

Zap!

Poof!

Maybe you don't even realize it, but you're building superpowers, too. That's another reason I wrote this book: To help you realize just how strong you are already. It's amazing what you'll accomplish when you start pulling out the tools whenever you need them.

This book is about finding out who you really are, how much you trust yourself, and what you truly believe you can do.

I've boiled down all of the lessons I've learned into what I think of as the seven superpowers of personal transformation. I've lived them and used them, and I want you to build and use yours as well.

You and I probably have a lot more in common than you think. If you pay attention to what went down with Shaun T, you'll get some ideas about how to bring about your own happily-ever-afters, too.

Let's run through the inventory of the *T Is for Transforma-*

tion superpowers that can help you survive the zigs and accelerate through the zags.

In order to advance, it helps to be . . .

UNCOMFORTABLE: Wait. What? Life begins at the end of your comfort zone. And that's fine, if you're willing to plan for and take smart risks.

FULL OUT: Here's your force multiplier—the enthusiasm, excitement, and commitment you put into every plan that can drive you forward.

CREATIVE: You can find (or make!) the tools you need to cut your way out of personal traps, and you can identify helping hands that can lift you up.

FLEXIBLE: You can swerve through the twists and turns, and accelerate through changes to reach for the life you really want.

SELFISH: That's right. Shaun T is giving you permission to be the center of your universe, but in a *good* way.

FEELIN' IT: You identify your passions and feel them all the way, because that's ultimately what determines success.

BANANAS: When you're pushing your life forward, there are bound to be surprises, disappointments, eye-openers, and other WTF moments. Plan for them, accept them, enjoy them, learn from them, and move forward because of them

I know you can make these seven superpowers work in your life and bring incredible change. How do I know that? Because I did it. And I wouldn't ask you to try anything that hasn't worked for me, first.

Starting after Chapter Five, you'll find ways to test your superpowers, plus specific exercises that will help you practice using them.

Ready? Press "Play" on the next awesome phase of your life.

CHAPTER TWO

MY BLACK BUDDY

The struggle always comes before the happy ending. In fact, you could make the case that without struggle, there are no happy endings—or even happy middles or beginnings.

TRUTHBOMB: Just like the frog always comes before the prince, the wound comes before the healing.

So, let's look at what has gone down for *you* so far. You've probably had some successes worth remembering, but there have probably also been some painful periods that you would just as soon forget.

But, if you don't understand the hurt, if you don't take the time to make sense of why you felt the way you did, you're unlikely to heal going forward.

That's how this chapter begins. You may want to cover your eyes at some points, but what 8-year-old Shaun Thompson went through was the necessary first step on a journey that led him to where he is today.

He's the one who gave me the strength to choose the path that I'm on, rather than having a disastrous path chosen for me by the worst person in my life.

As you read my story, think about your own. Whatever went down, the more clear-eyed you are about your past, the sharper the vision you can bring to your future.

THERE WERE ANGRY FORCES PUSHING AND pulling at my house when I was growing up, and it felt like it all might come crashing down on me. From a very early age, I turned a hard shell against the world to protect myself. When I started day-care, I was the little kid who grabbed onto his momma's leg at drop-off time, screaming like they were about to throw me into the fire instead of a classroom. I was like, *"I hate these people. I'm not going to play with nobody. Take me home right now!"*

In my confusion and vulnerability, I built defenses: I refused to speak with anybody but my brother Ennis and my mom, and I hid within the four walls of my closet, where I spent most of my time. That's right, I was in the closet before I even knew what being in the closet was all about.

At least I had a friend in there.

In fact, to know about me as a little kid, you need to meet a toddler-size black doll with kinky hair and a hard, plastic head. He was My Black Buddy, and he was my only true friend for the first decade of my life. I'm lucky my mom bought him for me, because without him, I had nobody.

I'd spend hours in a make-believe world with him, cutting and combing his hair, telling him stories, and, when necessary, using his hard, plastic head as a weapon against intruders. Even my brother felt the blows. (Sorry for the bruises, Ennis!) I was desperate for somebody to protect me, somebody to stick by me, somebody to occupy my mind. It's pathetic that I could only find it in a child-size doll, but at least I had that. My Black Buddy seemed like one of the only friends I could count on in a world where the people closest to me either did me harm or failed to protect me from it.

Can you imagine me as a world-hating, hostile little kid?

The same guy who now hugs everybody, who works out with 20,000 people at a time during a Beachbody Summit? Sometimes, I have a hard time connecting those dots, too.

But as I look back, I can see how each step—backward or forward—was critical to my arrival where I am today. Life is relentless: You make one choice, gauge results, make another, and then a little piece of chaos knocks you sideways. But all of that adds to your experience, teaches you lessons, and maybe furnishes a new superpower or two. If you're paying attention, and harvesting the fruits of your experience, you *can* move forward. I have done that, and I want nothing more than to help it happen for you, too.

If you feel stuck, maybe it's because you have tools you're not using or lessons you're not applying. Transformation comes from correcting both of those things, but you have to will yourself into action. I did that after some serious blows that life dealt to me. But I learned to hit back. I know you can, too.

But change didn't come quickly for me. In the early days, I needed My Black Buddy for defense, because there were others in my life who were an immediate danger.

I spent the first 7 years of my life in a one-room apartment on Baltimore Avenue in West Philadelphia. My earliest memory is of my mom washing me in a yellow basin in the kitchen sink, which was in the living room, which was the hallway to the dark bathroom—a closet, more like—and the only bedroom as well.

Everything back then seemed huge to me—those high stairs up to the apartment, the park across the street, the crumbling porch wall my older brother Ennis fell off of one time. But, when I go back there now, the place looks tiny; our apartment was probably less than 400 square feet for two adults and two kids. And I see a struggling family trying to make it in an apartment where we could barely breathe.

It's not that we lacked oxygen; the rattling window frames

let in plenty of that. But we were suffocating from the lies we told about our lives together. My mom tried hard, wanting the best for us. Most of my very best traits come from her—my openness to change, my way of reaching out to people, my way of bouncing back from a tough blow. But she turned to the wrong men for comfort and companionship.

I never knew my biological father.

I've heard stories about how my mom moved to Louisiana to be with this guy. They had twin boys together—Ennis and Eric. My mom was awakened at 5:00 a.m. on July 18th, 1977, by my brother screaming in the crib. She jumped out of bed, from a deep sleep, to run to the crib. That's when she discovered Eric, the brother I never met, cold and stiffening in the crib. The cause: sudden infant death syndrome (SIDS), and his absence haunts all of us to this day.

My mom was 21 at the time.

Her grief, and the fear that went with it, might explain some of the questionable men she accepted into her life, and mine. She fought a lot with my biological father, but in the meantime, she got pregnant with me. During one of those fights, he pushed her out of a bathroom window.

We were both lucky to survive that fall.

She left him with me still in utero, and Ennis just a year old, and moved closer to her family. She was alone when I was born in Camden, New Jersey, across the river.

She brought me home to an inner-city apartment, grieving the loss of a child, reeling from an abusive relationship, and with a 1-year-old and a new baby. She needed warmth and support. And the man she chose was even worse for our little family than the last guy. He joined our family when I was 2 years old—the only father I ever knew. So, I was part of a two-parent household, but I put that in *huge* air quotes.

He wasn't a stepfather.

A step*monster* is more like it.

Before the people in my family understood who this guy

really was, they kind of looked up to him. Okay, he was a violent alcoholic, but at least he hung in there with my mom. He could keep a job, and his money helped the family move up the ladder and out of Philly.

Maybe I saw him a little more clearly than most. Even from early on.

I can remember kneeling on the couch in our living room, which was backed up against the windows in the front of our apartment building. From that lookout, I could see our neighborhood and find out what my neighbors were up to.

One time, I saw him doing a West Philly version of *Fight Club*, trading punches with another man across the street. Who knows what that was about? Maybe a manhood contest, marking territory, or just the fun of a random head whomping. There was blood, and bone cracking, and an animal fury unlike I've ever seen anywhere outside of an MMA cage fight.

After a while, the fight broke up, the winner and loser (or two big losers) disengaged. Soon after, I heard footsteps on the stairs. The stepmonster appeared in the door, beaten and bloody, and stepped over to the kitchen sink to wash up, fouling the same place my mom washed me as a baby. Then, he went back into the street for round two. Something seriously wrong with *that*.

His battlefield wasn't confined to the street outside my window, either.

Another early memory is of riding in the backseat of our battered car, and my mom and the stepmonster yelling at each other up front. Ennis and I were taking it all in, wide-eyed, scared silent for once. We stopped at a red light, and the stepmonster bolted from the car. Naturally, in our crazy world, my mom went after him.

So, there's Ennis and me, alone on the street in a car with no adults, winter wind blowing through open doors, my mom and this guy laying into each other on the sidewalk, horns honking all around us.

Two-parent household, my ass. More like a three-ring circus, with an evil clown for a ringmaster.

I remember thinking, at the time: *This is crazy. I'm cold, and I might die. Why are Ennis and me in this car all alone? What's going to happen to us?*

The stepmonster was good for one thing, at least: dealing with rodents.

He used to set traps—snap!—and toss the dead carcasses. Perfect job for him, in fact.

Except one time, he decided to have a little fun with Shauny, instead.

I remember I was in the bath, enjoying the warm water and bubbles and that clean soapy smell, when the stepmonster entered the bathroom. He was holding something in his hand, and I didn't realize what it was immediately. He walked over, crouched next to the tub, extended his hand, and thrust a dead, squashed mouse toward my penis.

He must have enjoyed my shrieking and the geyser of bathwater that erupted.

Painful memories for me, yes. Maybe you have some like that. I couldn't blame you if you are reluctant to pull them out and examine them. It has taken me years to reach peace with the feelings that that scared little boy in the backseat had. But I promise you: Unless you are able to look your former self in the eye, comfort your younger self, and once and for all accept that chapter in the past, you will keep living the pain every day. The deeper it's buried, the more urgently it needs to rise up to the surface and be acknowledged and understood. Only then can you convert it into a superpower that you can apply to similar circumstances in the future.

Yes, I was alone and frightened in the car that day. But it helped me learn to seek the right kinds of relationships, and make sure I could grab the steering wheel when I needed to. So, my current life wouldn't be possible if it hadn't happened to me.

IF ANY LITTLE KID EVER HAD a reason to believe that it was a mean world, that people weren't to be trusted, it was little Shauny. At least I was in the craziness with Ennis, who wasn't crazy at all.

As I grew up, I followed my big brother Ennis around like a little baby duck. We would dress alike; both of us had big old Afros even as little tiny kids; and I signed up for every activity he did. I wasn't avoiding the shadow of my older brother, I *was* his shadow.

For all the weird stuff that went down during my childhood, my brother Ennis was my only normal relationship. Okay, yes, we had our disagreements. We competed at everything, but we were so close, and he felt like home to me, at least for my first 14 years.

It's sad and funny now for me to think about my two pillars of support, back then: One real, one imaginary. I was desperate, of course, but at least I could sort out the friends—Ennis and My Black Buddy—from the enemy stepmonster. A little later in the book, I'll take you through an exercise that will help you divide your home team from the opposition, but for now, ask yourself a few questions:

Who are my true pillars of support, and who is ready to tear me down if I step out of line?

Whose path should I follow, and who is ready to lead me someplace that I don't want to go?

Who's a positive example, and who's a negative one?

When you sort out the Ennises from the evildoers, the Buddies from the bad blood, you'll begin to build a support network that can catch you when you're falling, and launch you when you're ready to fly.

I WAS AN EXTRAORDINARILY SENSITIVE LITTLE boy. Everything I felt, I felt 100 percent. I was that kid that, if we went to the Jersey Shore, I would be walking 30 feet behind my family because . . . the lights! The ocean! The clothes! It was sensory overload. My mom bought one of those kid leashes to link onto 4-year-old me, or else I may have wandered off permanently.

The stepmonster interpreted "slow walker" as "mentally slow," so he called me Turtle. I was so far behind everybody else that I was more reptile than human, you see. But even then, I knew: I was slow because the world was awesome. If I sped up, I might miss something great. I wanted to take it all in. Especially before I learned to reach out to people, I had to keep a lot going on inside to fill up my time, my life, and my overactive brain. I was good company for me, and I had to be!

I may not have been sharing much with the outside world, but I had an active inner life. I know now that I was taking it all in: the bad and the good. It's one of the reasons I so appreciate little Shauny when I look back at him now. He was biding his time, observing the world, preparing to advance with the best people and activities, and leave behind the worst.

I hope you'll give yourself a break with this, as well: Just because you haven't taken steps yet toward that new job, or away from that old relationship, doesn't mean you can't or won't. You may just be in your own "slow walking" phase, watching carefully in anticipation of the moment when you have learned enough to succeed brilliantly.

At least the stepmonster got one part of it right with my nickname: I needed a hard shell to protect me, and growing up, I doubted it would ever be safe to poke my head out of it.

When it was time for us to enroll in school, my mom pulled a fast one, and shifted us into a stronger district. She informed the school board of Deptford, New Jersey—about

8 miles away, where my grandparents lived—that we were residents, and enrolled us.

Every school day, she would roust Ennis and me out of bed at 5:00 a.m. We would stagger down to her beat-up black car, with a brown door and a faulty starter. I remember thinking: Why doesn't anybody else drive a car like this? It was the first sign I had that we were barely scraping by.

But I give my mom credit: She was trying to work it out for us.

She'd crank that dead engine until it coughed and wheezed to life, and rev the engine to warm the car up beyond icebox level. Then, we'd make the trek over to my grandparents' house via the Walt Whitman bridge. And *then*, we'd stand in front of Mom-Mom and Pop-Pop's house to catch the school bus to Lake Tract Elementary School.

Our school commute ended when my mom got a better-paying job, and we were able to upgrade to a neighborhood about a mile from where Mom-Mom and Pop-Pop lived. After the move, we had a whole house to ourselves, and school was a quick bus ride away. I was *so* happy: *Oh, my God*, I thought. *I got my own room! We actually have stairs and a driveway! And a basement!*

On the surface, things were looking good. Of course, that's the problem with the surface. It's like a frozen pond. With a glossy layer of ice, you don't see the dark layer of muck down below.

IS IT ANY WONDER I WENT looking for escape routes? In school, we had a reading program called The Super Kids. The main characters drove around having adventures in a school bus; it was designed to teach us how far reading could take us in life. I loved to read, and I loved those kids, and maybe I was looking for magical transportation that would take me any-where beyond the closet. My stepmonster wasn't going to do that for me, and my mom was just too exhausted from work and dealing with Ennis and me. So, naturally, I turned to my grandparents, the Reverend Charles Dawson, and his wife, Effie, aka Pop-Pop and Mom-Mom.

If my home life was all dysfunction and chaos, theirs was calm and harmony. They loved me, and I knew it. So, when I said, "Pop-Pop, would you make a bus out of cardboard and bring it to school?" he didn't hesitate.

Okay, I'm sure they had to call my teacher and say, "Shaun needs a *what*, made out of *what*?"

But, here's everything you need to know about my Pop-Pop: He did it.

I can still remember him dragging the big boxes into my classroom, helping us decorate it like the Super Kids school bus, all my kindergarten classmates playing in it, and me as proud as I could be that *my* grandfather made it, and knowing that he did it for *me*.

THE STORY OF MY CHILDHOOD GETS a lot darker than it was in that closet with My Black Buddy, but still I say: I love that little kid, and I credit him for all he did to launch me into a life I love.

Life is unfair. People can be cruel. Each of us has been hurt, and each of us has suffered things that we did nothing to bring about. None of that changes for any of us, no matter how we choose to look at our lives. *What changes is how we react to it.*

Every one of us is hiding in some kind of closet, whether it's an abusive person in our past or present, a memory of past failures, or a struggle to get the resources that we need. But by packing that mess away into some dark secret place, you are limiting your access to the best part of your life ahead.

We're gonna break out together, if you'll just give it a try.

If you built a closet, know that the four high walls aren't real. You've imagined them into existence, and you can tear them down just as easily as you built them, by deciding they're flimsier than you imagined, or that they don't exist at all.

Your mind is a sledgehammer. Swing it!

CHAPTER THREE

LEARNING
HOW
TO BREATHE

Take a look at the turning points in your life.

The moments when you were suffering, or just dissatisfied, and then decided you wouldn't live like that anymore.

The afternoon you quit that job you hated.

The night you told that lame boyfriend to "bleep" off.

The time you looked in the mirror and didn't recognize who you'd become, and vowed to make a change.

The drink you threw down the sink, or the cigarettes you dumped into the toilet.

The morning you dropped the doughnut, laced up your running shoes, and went out for a run.

Turning points can feel like your very best moments, or your very worst, but they have one thing in common: They separate out your life into a before and an after, and they are like beacons of light pointing out the events that caused everything in your life to be different.

Sometimes, it feels like that's when the transformation happens. But really, your life leading up to moments is a series of small successes (or failures), and your life after that moment or moments is a series of choices on where to head next. Down or up?

Your mission: Start looking back at those moments, learning what brought them about, and pull the levers that bring about positive change.

I DIDN'T START LIVING UNTIL I was 14 years old.

I was born in 1978, but it took me until 1992 to decide that I wouldn't be the victim in my life story. I chose to live for myself, rather than suffer through what others were doing to me. My first 14 years could have turned me toward the darkness for the rest of my life. If I was looking for reasons to hide or reasons to hate, they were everywhere as I grew up.

I wouldn't wish my years of scared silence on anybody. But as bad as it was, it set me on the journey I'm still on today. So many times, when a disappointment comes now, or a relationship goes bad, or a lawyer-scammer-businessperson tries to get the jump on me in a deal, I just repeat my mantra: "I have survived the worst parts of my journey already, and there is nothing the world can throw at me that I can't handle. I just need to be as strong *today* as little Shauny was so many years ago."

Everything I needed to learn about facing hurdles—how to be real with myself, how to be honest with others, how to take charge of my life—I learned from my 14-year-old self. He's my hero, because he was strong enough to seize control of himself and his future.

Sexual abuse is a curse. You're about to read how it happened to me.

TRUTHBOMB: Dealing with the worst that can happen can prepare you to chase the best that can happen for the rest of your life.

I didn't have a choice or a voice in what happened back in my childhood. But when I was ready, I responded.

I still can.

I still do.

Do you?

SOCIAL WORKERS AND CHILD PSYCHOLOGISTS KNOW to look for a haunted silence as a potential sign of abuse. Nobody saw or understood that in me. I just hid away in my closet and waited to see if anybody would notice I was missing or hurting or in trouble.

Mostly, they didn't.

Or, maybe they were afraid of what they might find if they asked questions. The urge to turn away is powerful, and I get that. I've long ago forgiven the people who could have stepped in to save me, but didn't.

Either way, the stepmonster took full advantage. I was alone, and ripe for the taking.

I wasn't an easy kid, as I've said.

Because of the walls I built around myself, nobody could see into my life. The stepmonster was counting on that when he chose me as his victim. The worse the abuse got, the quieter I got.

He kept me off-balance, confused, frightened. When he approached me quietly, with strokes rather than threats, with kindness instead of a dead mouse, it felt like I'd escaped something even worse. That was his plan, and he executed it perfectly.

The abuse began after our move to Deptford.

The basement there was the stepmonster's lair; I don't think my mom ever went down there, probably under threat. He kept his porn stash down there, lying around in plain sight. As a little kid, I knew that wasn't meant for me, and I averted my eyes. And I didn't feel good about it when he announced that we were going down there for "movie night," one time when my cousin was over.

It started out okay. We were watching a movie, sharing popcorn, just like a family would. But, at some point, the step-monster invented some task for my cousin and sent him upstairs, to get him out of the room for a while.

Then, he turned his attention to me.

"Shaun," he asked, "Have you ever kissed a man before? Have you ever kissed anyone?"

"No," I said, swallowing hard. I was 8 years old.

"Well, I'm going to show you."

It didn't go beyond that . . . the first time. As if a grown man tongue-kissing a young boy wasn't bad enough. He must have been waiting to hear if I'd squawk. Call him out. Complain to my mom. Instead, I was ashamed, so I was silent. If anybody would avoid speaking about the unspeakable, it was silent Shauny.

It was just the opening he was looking for.

There was a pattern to the abuse.

He would come home drunk on weekend nights.

He'd pick a fight with my mother in the kitchen to get her out of the way. Then, the coast was clear for what would come next.

He'd come upstairs, close the bathroom door, and turn on the light to make her think that he was in there. That's when he'd sneak into my bedroom. He'd start out by rubbing my butt, then flip me over. He'd perform oral sex on me.

I know now that it wasn't about sex, it was about power. And he had all of it.

Many nights, I'd drift off to sleep, and in my dream, I was in wonderland. An amazing feeling was coming over my body. And then, I'd become aware of the stench of alcohol, the scrape of bristles on my bare skin. And I would awaken to find I was being molested.

I went from pure pleasure to total terror: *I don't think this is supposed to be happening to me*, I would think to myself, digging my fingers into the mattress. *I don't think this is right.*

The stepmonster had attempted anal rape the first night he molested me in my bedroom, but even he realized that I was too little to survive a penetration without major trauma. Not that he cared about me particularly, but if he'd gone ahead, it would have provided *evidence* of what he was doing to me. So, he worked me over in other ways. Getting himself off by getting me off.

But as a result of that attempted assault on my anus, I was constantly clenching my sphincter against any potential intruder. My brother Ennis remembers that, as a little kid, I didn't poop—like, *ever*.

Weird, right? Uncomfortable. Unnatural.

It was all of that, every waking moment of my life. But it was especially humiliating for me during the championship game in my Pee Wee football league. I was one of my team's best players, but, on game day, I could barely move on the field because of what was building up inside me. There are some things that you can't hold back forever. Finally, the dam broke while I waited for kickoff, and I soiled myself in my uniform.

Could there be a more embarrassing experience for a 10-year-old kid?

I was covered in mud from the field, so the load didn't show through my uniform. But after the game, I suffered through the longest ride of my life, fearing that I'd stink up the team bus and be called out for crapping myself like a toddler. I made it home, finally, and buried the soiled underpants deep in my brother's closet. What a mystery that provoked, when the filthy evidence was discovered years later.

Okay, laugh at me if you like. But I ask: What do you have buried in your closet, too shameful to pull out?

There's something, right?

Will you deal, or continue to conceal?

At 8 years old, I gave in to him. He was a man, I was a child. I couldn't run to Ennis, who was sleeping five steps away from my bedroom, and tell him this was happening to me. I didn't have the power to run downstairs and tell my mom that her no-good man was molesting me. For the next 4 years of my life, I went to bed terrified.

But fear wasn't the *only* thing I felt.

This is just one of the difficult aspects of abuse: An adult enters the life of a vulnerable child, and gives him something nobody else does. The closeness. The focus. The attention. It makes him feel special . . . at a terrible cost.

So I absorbed the worst thing that my stepmonster could deliver and thought I was protecting my family by doing so. He was so unpredictable. Kind to my mom one moment, cruel the next. Giving me special treatment, then turning on me, then giving me "special treatment" of a sexual kind.

He kept all of us off-balance, so that if he was actually behaving like a human being, we were grateful. The sense of dread and confusion was so great that, one time, my mom gathered Ennis and me together to ask *our* advice: "Should I stay with him, or should we leave?"

She was asking *us*? Her little *kids*?

It shows me how badly she was up against it, as well.

Against this backdrop of abuse and confusion, I didn't want to do anything that would throw my stepmonster into a rage. If he was attacking me, there was less venom to spend on the rest us, right?

I'd like to say that I acted heroically to stop my stepmonster's abuse. Created a scene. Accused my attacker. Sent him packing.

None of that happened.

My approach was that, if I wasn't ready to say anything about it (and I wasn't) or do anything to end it (and I couldn't), then I had to accept it. So, I did.

Everybody in my family had a role to fill and a job to do. Mom worked. Ennis got straight A's. I was abused.

It was a dark secret I had to keep, because I knew it was evil. *When I let it happen, without complaining to anybody, it became my fault, too.*

How wrong is that? On how many levels?

I hated the stepmonster. But his actions were candy-coated—like the way rat poison tastes good to the rat. My abuse was laced with pleasure, and the excitement a child feels when he is chosen for something nobody else receives. Or can know about.

Secrets are exciting to a kid. Even devastating ones.

No wonder I kept to myself: Everybody has nightmares; mine happened when I was awake.

But during those years there was a counterbalance in my life, as well.

I can picture the front of my first-grade classroom just as if I were sitting in my little-kid desk right now. There was the chalkboard, and above it ran the alphabet. Next to that, a little monkey, who taught me my right hand from my left. And next to *that*, a scroll with my first TRUTHBOMB spelled out in beautiful script:

THE GOLDEN RULE "Do unto others as you would have them do unto you."

Those ancient words exist in various forms in all the world's major religions. But they were new to me, and they gave me a whole new way of relating to people.

Oh, my gosh, I thought, hopefully, *if I'm nice to people, they're gonna be nice to me?*

Notice that I stated it, even to myself, as a question, especially after the abuse began.

No trust. No belief. But I could hope it would be true, and search it out in my own life.

Sometimes, the simplest truths are ones that are easiest to move right on past without noticing. Yeah, yeah, today you think, *do unto others . . . blah, blah, blah. I've heard that, now what's up on Twitter since the last time I checked 2 minutes ago? What snarky comments are people tweeting or retweeting?*

But, is there anything else you need to know about how to get along with people?

I had a long way to go before the Golden Rule could really take over in my own life.

It became more like, do unto Shaun before somebody catches you and throws you in jail for child endangerment.

So, yes, there's a flip side to the Golden Rule. You can do right by people, and trust you'll receive the same in return, or you can wrong them miserably, repeatedly, and pass suffering down the generations.

The stepmonster made his choice.

I'd have to make mine.

Have you made yours?

YOU'VE HEARD OF THE LION THAT has been so completely trained that it won't leave its cage even when the door is accidentally left open? That was me for the first 14 years of my life. But a series of incidents finally woke up enough rage and hurt inside of me to motivate me out into the world.

The first happened when I was 12 years old and showing signs of being a scientific brainiac. All the super-nerds were aware of the Edmund Scientific Corporation, a supplier of geeky gear to junior Einsteins. Put Shauny down in that corner, complete with the fluffy hair.

I was planning an ambitious science-fair project, and the stepmonster promised that he would take me to Edmund Scientific, in a neighboring town, one Saturday morning to get the supplies I needed. But for this favor, I had to pay his price: a sexual one. I was used to the routine now—a chore I did to get what I needed from this demon who haunted our house.

But, after he had taken his pleasure that day, he didn't hold up his end of the bargain. He backed out on his promise to take me to Edmund Scientific. And because the molestation happened in the daylight this time, I had to actually *see* what he was doing.

I felt disgusted, but that disgust was followed by anger: He broke the ugly agreement that we had, and that broke something else inside of me. So, the Edmund Scientific Corporation, finally, convinced me to begin planning my escape.

Around this time, he pulled away, too. I'd done an unforgivable thing for a sex toy: I'd entered puberty. When I was no longer a child, he was no longer sexually excited by me.

Sick, on a whole new level.

His nighttime visits ended. He didn't even look at me anymore.

But, to show you how bad it had gotten, I felt that the abuse had given me a certain status. It wasn't happening to anybody else I knew—or at least, that they could talk about. I'd been conditioned to accept his sexual advances, so I wasn't prepared when they stopped suddenly.

In the strangest way, I had been abandoned, and it hurt.

I kept this hidden in my closet for a long time, even into my adult life. But, I am so glad that I finally understood this part of my story. Wrong as his sexual attentions were, they made me feel special. Sometimes that's true about sex, even horribly wrong sex.

The thing that hurt me most was that as afraid and unsafe and unhappy as it had made me, physically, *it felt good.* After it stopped, I tried to entice him again. I would stand in my room in my underwear with my back facing the door, so he could see.

In my head, I was asking, *why don't you want me anymore?*

While most people have their hearts broken in their teens because of a first boyfriend or girlfriend, I had my heart broken by my abuser. How screwed up does that sound? Since I had this breakthrough in understanding my abuse, I've learned that this is actually a common reaction. It's yet another painful reality that abuse survivors need to come to terms with in order to finally heal. Because I have been able to open up the closet and face this, I am no longer ashamed of what happened to me, and I am no longer ashamed of how I felt about it. I can face all of those things now, and I'm stronger for it. That was the truth I needed to reflect on and learn to accept.

Although I couldn't process that truth at the time, I knew it was time for me to finally act: I needed to leave the house where the abuser lived, even if it meant leaving my mom and Ennis, too.

So, I developed an escape plan.

Mom-Mom and Pop-Pop's house was just a mile away, but they might as well have been living on Mars. My home was my longtime torture chamber; theirs was a safe haven.

I planned my getaway in detail. I had to act at just the right time, and I had to be careful not to make it seem like I was threatening to leave my family. No dramatics; the last thing I wanted to do was call out my stepmonster and give him a reason to slam the door on my jail cell.

Or kill somebody.

I needed the path of least resistance, and I found it one summer afternoon when my grandmother drove by my mom's house for a visit. Mom-Mom never got out of the car when she visited; she didn't want to be in the house with the stepmonster, either.

When she rolled up, I saw my chance. I headed out to the road, and she rolled down her window.

"Mom-Mom," I began, "Do you think I could come live with you and Pop-Pop for high school?"

She didn't express surprise or push me away. She simply asked, "Why?"

I had my reason ready: "I'd be really good at helping around the house."

Since when are 14-year-olds good at helping around the house—unless we're talking about helping themselves to seconds of Mom-Mom's famous scrambled eggs?

But my grandmother didn't blink an eye. She just told me that I'd have to ask my mother, who was just then stepping out onto the front steps of the house.

I didn't risk putting it as a question.

Instead, I made a statement that changed my life: "I'm going to live with Mom-Mom and Pop-Pop," I told her, "because *they need me.*"

My mom quietly accepted my proposal, just like Mom-Mom had.

That I would even *choose* to leave must have said more than my simple proposal had. That both had agreed to my escape plan *without any discussion* tells me that they knew, or suspected, exactly why I needed to make this break.

MY FIRST NIGHT AT MY GRANDPARENTS' house, I got into bed, closed my eyes, and realized: I did it. I escaped.

Then, I started crying.

These weren't quiet tears of joy. They were gushing tears, cleansing tears, tears that washed away the guilt and hurt from 4 years of sexual abuse. The dam burst. The floods came.

I wasn't quiet about it, either. This was a celebration, after all.

Mom-Mom and Pop-Pop heard my crying and burst into my room. They asked me, "What's wrong? Why are you crying? Do you want to go back home?"

My response must have made them wonder. Or, maybe it just confirmed what they already suspected.

"No," I told them. "I'm so happy. I'm just so happy."

My grandfather did what came natural at that point: He knelt down next to my bed and prayed over me.

I fell asleep to the sound of his whispered prayers.

It's such a kid reaction: conking out while the grown-ups are doing their adult thing. But it means so much to me now to think of 14-year-old Shaun drifting off. After a lifetime of nightmare bedside visits, I could finally sleep in peace.

The next morning, I awoke, realized where I was, and said aloud: "This is my life!"

I could breathe free at last.

MY GRANDFATHER, AS A PREACHER, WAS always talking about being born again, about accepting Jesus Christ as your personal savior. Well, at that moment, Mom-Mom and Pop-Pop were my saviors, and I was truly reborn.

Finally, I was free to live my own life as Shaun, rather than suffering as somebody's victim. Nobody rescued me. I made a plan, executed it, and rescued *myself*.

That's how I know that you can do the same.

TRUTHBOMB: Stay a victim, and you grant power to the person who victimized you.

No way did the stepmonster deserve to have that power over me. It took time, but I found a way to take the power back for myself, and I'm still running on the energy that doing so gave me.

Not everyone is abused physically, thank goodness. But at some point or another, almost everybody has the experience of being a victim to someone else's cruelty. Some people grant that power to others their whole lives, even after the abuser has left the crime scene. If you stay silent, they're still in charge, still abusing you. But once you refuse to be a victim, you seize the power for yourself. That's when *you* . . . *f*ing* . . . *win*.

It's transformation time.

CHAPTER FOUR

THE RULE OF SEVEN

S elfishness gets a bad rap.

You hear people say, "she only thinks of herself," or "he acts like the whole world revolves around him," and it's pretty much always in a negative context. I'm here to say: You need to do exactly that, sometimes.

If I hadn't left my mother and brother behind when I escaped the stepmonster, I doubt whether I'd be talking to you right now. I had to act to save my life, even though it meant leaving two of the people I loved most in the world. Maybe you need to, too, even if you're not up against a threat like I was.

We all have people who depend on us: a wife or husband, kids, employees on the job, maybe an aging parent or two. I'm not talking about abandoning any of them with a me-first attitude. What I am saying is that if you're not taking care of yourself, then you're not going to be able to really help anybody else, either.

If you're the sun, then the planets aren't going to benefit if you flame out. You've heard the expression: If momma ain't happy, ain't nobody happy. Well, I'd like to adapt that: If you ain't happy, ain't nobody in your circle happy, either.

Is it selfish to have a dream? Make a plan and execute it? No.

Is it selfish to take steps—get a master's degree, see a counselor, schedule gym time—to realize those dreams? I repeat: No.

That's called striving to be the best person you can be in order to better enrich the lives of the people you love. It's what you do to make sure that you're broadcasting light and heat to all the "planets" that are counting on it. Burn on!

And that means be selfish, because all the people in your life will benefit if you are. You get more of what you need in your life, and you'll have more to share around. (Later on in the book, I'll take you through an exercise to build selfishness. But, if you just can't wait, turn to page 204, to start being the center of your own world, for a change.)

MY LIFE, FROM AGE 14 TO 21, is when I was reborn. I went from making my sacrifice—absorbing abuse so my family could be safe—to finding what I wanted and could be good at.

I could have sent out birth announcements, that's how "brand new" I felt. I fell asleep one night with my grandfather praying over me, and when I woke up the next morning, my eyes opened like a new chapter in a book. The old one was finished, and I wasn't going back.

I mean literally.

The negative energy blowing through the hallways of my mom's house exploded me into new mental space. That can work for you too, you know. You can take the energy of a negative situation and let that blow you out of that space and into a whole new one. Think Dorothy and the tornado: The spinning power of it threw her and Toto all the way to Oz, where she found Technicolor, cool red shoes, Glinda the Good Witch, and a powerful wizard. You'll never get there if you hang back in Kansas.

TRUTHBOMB: You can ride the tornado! Let it blow you as far away as possible from your dark, stormy place!

When you find yourself struggling, I urge you to gauge the energy in the room. If it's tornado-alley negative, that means it's strong enough blow you straight over the rainbow when you're ready.

First, though, you need to separate yourself from that negative. Put the funnel cloud at arm's length, and realize that just because it's dark and swirling, doesn't mean that you have to be, too. Instead, use the spinning force to lift you up to a new place.

Use your anger to motivate you.

Use your fear to put an adrenaline kick into your sprint.

See the negative force, and match it with a positive power *that you generate within you.* You are capable of creating your own weather system, and it will blow you where you need to go.

My situation forced me to make incredibly hard choices—should I stay at home with my brother and mother, or should I do the selfish thing and get myself away from my abuser?

Should I risk exposure by asking to leave the house, or keep my mouth shut and stay in the house so that I wouldn't have to tell anybody why I had to leave?

It took a long time, but I got to a point where the negative energy was so strong that I was forced to make a call about what I was willing to endure and what I wasn't. And for me, that meant escaping my house at all costs.

Maybe you've been in a position where you feel like you're faced with an impossible choice: Ending a marriage that's not good for you even if it means disrupting the lives of your children; leaving a job you need because the team of people around you is too difficult; changing up a couch-bound lifestyle for something healthier, even though your family is on that couch with you.

When you've been immersed in negative energy for a long time, you may feel like there's no escape, but trust me: The tornado *is* your escape. Every day, you have a choice about how you live, and you can choose whether the negativity is a fair trade-off for some balancing positives. If it's not, then it's time to start looking toward Oz.

Let the tornado move you, like it moved me.

Not that my break was a clean one, necessarily.

Looking back now, I can see that I left home and just stashed my emotional baggage in the dark recesses of the basement. Eventually, I'd have to go back to unpack it for good, and that meant talking to a shrink about it for 5 years. (Yes, I highly recommend that you seek help when it's time to start really digging into your past. Some burdens are too heavy to lift on your own.) But right at that moment, 14-year-old Shaun needed to keep his eyes forward, and that's what he did.

PLANET SHAUN WENT FROM ORBITING A black hole to revolving around the blazing sun itself. I'm talking here about my Pop-Pop, who—true confession—wasn't actually my grandfather at all. (My family has a way of doing things the most complicated way possible.) My mom's biological parents started having kids when her dad was around 30 and her mom was a teenager, and it was a very reproductive union. They couldn't handle all of those kids, so they started farming them out to other families. My mom ended up living with her aunt and uncle, who were childless; when Ennis and I came along, we naturally thought of my mom's aunt and uncle as our grandparents—Mom-Mom and Pop-Pop—because my mom thought of them as her parents.

Got all that? Good!

It couldn't have worked out better. They cherished us as if we were their own biological grandchildren and provided an example of love and stability in a world that had too little of that for my first 14 years.

As a young man, my Pop-Pop was a state-champion boxer, and I picked up some of my own instincts as a battler from him. He eventually laid down the gloves, picked up a Bible, and started fighting for people's souls.

One of the many souls he rescued was mine. I had a personal savior, and he was it.

When I moved into my grandfather's house, I was fully under his influence, and that meant church.

Lots and lots of church.

Wednesday night church.

Sunday all-day church.

Prayers before meals. Prayers after meals.

Prayers when I woke up. Prayers when I went to sleep. (Hey, it beats other kinds of bedside visits.)

I didn't resent it. This was life at their house, and if that's what it took to belong, I was all-in.

Some days, my grandfather would go to the farmers' market near where we lived and pick up day-old bread for cheap. Then, we'd drive into downtown Camden and deliver food to people who needed help. I'll always remember the looks on their faces. They were so grateful for his gift of bread—even day-old bread—to their families.

I'm not what you would call a traditionally religious person right now. The Golden Rule is enough for me. But I did pick up something in my grandfather's sermons. He knew how to heal people who were hurting.

I might have been shivering on those cold street corners and squirming on those hard church pews, but I was watching, listening, and learning, too. I saw his passion for what he did, and I wanted a piece of that in my life as well. Pop-Pop wasn't out on that street corner because he liked the sound of his own voice. He was using that powerful tool to reach into the lives of people who desperately needed change in their lives, but maybe had lost hope that they could ever pull that off. Living in a world with nothing but cold shoulders and short meals will do that to you.

And there was Pop-Pop with a loaf of bread and a message: I care about you, body and soul. And he meant every word of it, which is why his voice rang true and people listened to him. That bedrock authenticity was the reason why he could gather those needy souls into his arms and help them.

I didn't go into the ministry, but I speak with a passion that comes directly from Pop-Pop on the streets of Camden. I felt the hurt and found a way to heal, so I know every step in that process. That's where my voice comes from. When I tell somebody, "I know you can do this," I truly believe it, because I delivered the same message to myself in time to turn my life around.

I *so* want that for you, too.

Maybe you aren't desperate for the next loaf of bread, but you may be hurting just the same, and you need a source of hope in your life. Because Pop-Pop and others gave that to me, I'm on a life mission to pass it along to you as well—body and soul.

THE OTHER BIG INFLUENCE ON MY life at this time was sports. Ennis was already out on the football field, so, of course, the little baby duck followed him out there as well. I can remember riding over to the football field as a little kid, and Ennis got out and started walking toward practice. I took two steps and stopped. Big people were hitting each other out there!

"Mom, I'm not going to do that," I said, slamming the car door behind me. I didn't want to get stampeded on the gridiron.

But that wasn't my final decision.

The next season, I went to watch one of Ennis's games and discovered that it takes all kinds of kids to fill out a football roster. Some of them were actually 8-year-old-sized (i.e., equal to scrawny Shauny). So, I finally made it out onto the field with Ennis. I had my mishaps—like the one that ended up in my underwear—but sports gave me an outlet in which to grow stronger and try harder.

That's the way I was with sports as a kid and how I still operate today. I'm not one to throw myself out there and say, "I'll do whatever it takes to win," before I understand fully what the game is and what it will take for me to win it. I'm not sure anybody actually succeeds that way. Better to get back in the car if you have to, study up, and then commit, when you're ready.

It reminds me of how little "Turtle" used to trail along behind the family. You could say he wasn't making much progress. Or, you could say he was figuring out the best steps before he made his move.

You be the judge of it in your own life. If you're stagnating, that's no good. If you're studying, practicing, and building skills to prepare to get in the game, you're playing the right way. The winning way.

The biggest chase of my life came after I began to run track. The Deptford High School team was coached by Sonny Anderson, a state trooper with a bald head and a stern attitude.

It was just what I needed, in fact.

When I'm giving people some tough-trainer love in a class or on a DVD, I'm channeling Coach Anderson. He didn't care if you lapped a guy and were on pace for a world record. No smiles from him, just a set of instructions on how you could do it a little better next time.

A little better next time. An entire life of achievement can be built on those five little words. That's why I repeat them so often during workouts. Can you hang in there against exhaustion a few seconds longer? Can you complete five reps today when you did four yesterday?

TRUTHBOMB: Get a little better today than you were yesterday. Multiply that by 365 days in a year and your life will be transformed.

That process began for me at my first track practice, on March 6, 1992. We began with a mile run—under 6 minutes, no sweat—and then we did some drills: mummy kicks, high knees, side-to-side lunges, butt kicks. Then we got down and stretched a bit.

Hey, I thought, *track practice is easy! I'm ready for the showers.*

Then, Coach Anderson told us, "That was the warm-up. Now practice begins."

Anybody who has been through one of my *Shaun T Live* workouts has heard me echo that one. "Don't you go groaning at me!" I'll tell somebody in the crowd, who lets a complaint slip. "That was just the warm-up. We haven't even *begun* working yet!"

On the high-school track that day, Coach Anderson ordered us to complete eight 400-meter sprints with a 30-second rest in between. I had never even dreamed I could survive that, but it turned out—I could. Yes, my lungs were exploding, but I felt like something incredible was happening to me: I was being tested to see just how much I was capable of. This wasn't a time to show how much I could *comfortably* do; it was a question of how much I could do when I was already exhausted, sore, and *uncomfortable.*

TRUTHBOMB: The work doesn't begin until you get tired.

Coach was forcing me to dig deeper than I ever had before and to see what I was capable of when I stepped (okay, sprinted) outside of my comfort zone and then kept going. I had to ask: What was my core? Was I a jelly doughnut, or did I have stronger stuff inside?

I love doughnuts, but that gooey middle couldn't be the metaphor for my life. So, I started forging my iron core.

It was a revelation to me that I'll never forget. To this day, I love it when I surprise myself by pulling off something that I didn't know I could do.

Connecting with somebody who I thought was beyond my world, but finding out that we have a lot in common.

Or, moving into a scary, challenging space, and finding I belong there.

Think of a challenge in your own life—at work, at home, at the gym. I get it: It's scary because it seems hard. Another way to look at it is that it's exciting, because it's a chance to surprise yourself, and move your life into a whole new space. And here's the thing about a scary challenge: Once you tackle it, you gain superpowers that will help you face the next challenge, and the one after that.

If you dodge the challenge, it just sits there in your path, blocking forward progress. Don't let it!

It's one of the reasons I think that my at-home workouts are transformative for so many people: They provide a tough obstacle, plus the means to climb over it. People often say thank you to me for the workouts, but of course, they should just be thanking themselves. They did the work.

Faced with that challenge on the track, I came up with a strategy to overcome my weaknesses. I listened hard to what Coach was saying, and I put it into action. One day during practice, Coach Anderson told me that the last 70 meters is the most important part of the race, and if your arms are strong there, it's going to drive your knees high, and you're going to *go*.

So, what did I do?

Anybody who has done my *INSANITY* workouts knows how crazy I am about sprinting in place, with extreme arm pumping. It works your endurance, your big muscle groups, your abs, and your *mind*.

So, there I was, in the bathroom at age 16, full of testosterone and competitive fire, and I looked myself in the eye, in the mirror.

"How bad do you want it, Shaun?"

I would hit the stopwatch, sprint in place for 1 minute, pistoning my arms the whole time, take 30 seconds to gasp, and then sprint again. I did that 10 times in a row.

I hope nobody else needed to use that bathroom! (If they did, they probably heard all that pounding and gasping and thought: Better leave the teenager alone.)

I started making a habit of that exercise—looking myself in the mirror every time and challenging myself each time to do a little better than yesterday. The first race after my first round of bathroom workouts, my time was a little faster. The realization hit me hard: I put in the time and effort, and I saw the change in my results.

And it did work. I made it to the state championships in the 400-meter hurdles. But, what was really important was that I learned a step-by-step, skill-based approach to making myself better at the things I cared about. I wasn't going to make great leaps forward, so I committed to small hops instead. Burst from the starting blocks with precision. Practice the take-off for a hurdle until I nailed it. Run through the finish line, don't lean toward it. If I could master these skills one by one, they'd add up to making me a stronger competitor.

TRUTHBOMB: Concentrating on smaller victories makes the bigger ones more likely.

Many of the principles that carried me to my breakthrough with *INSANITY*, I first learned on the track.

The most important one:

TRUTHBOMB: The only thing holding you back is your own mind.

And there was another key lesson that Coach Anderson taught me as well. When we were exhausted, he asked for us to give a little (or sometimes a lot) more. And most of the time, it turned out that we could.

During those rare moments when I wasn't practicing or working, I'd be hanging around my hometown with friends. There was always one kid with a car, and it seemed like it always had less than a quarter-tank of gas. We'd scrounge under the seats and deep into our pockets for change to fill it up, but we always saw that needle dipping toward empty and beyond.

But we never ran out of gas.

Same thing on the track field in high school. No matter what drill Coach Anderson called out, and how far into the afternoon it was, and how much we hated to admit it, *we always found a reserve.*

Thanks for teaching me that, too, Coach Anderson.

Life is an exhausting track meet sometimes, and fate doesn't line up the events to give you a nice long rest in between sprints. But here's the deal: Usually, the only thing between you and a new sprint is deciding to throw yourself forward again. What your brain decides, your body will go along with.

It may be the ultimate superpower, in fact: Deciding that *you will move forward*, no matter what.

And finally, thanks Coach A, for choosing me (and Ennis!) to run the four-man relay. Great to be on my brother's team rather than trying to kick his ass all the time.

We spent countless hours practicing the hand-off: Watching my guy dash in and pound the baton into my hand, and then sprinting to carry it to the next runner. If you've watched Olympic track-and-field in your life—including the U.S. men's *and* women's teams—you've seen all the drops that end a relay team's chances in tears and heartbreak.

If you can't pass it, you ain't gonna win it.

In your life, you're constantly passing the baton . . . to *yourself*.

In a 4 x 100-meter dash, you have to hand it over in the passing zone or you're DQ'd. One runner blasts out of the gate, but, eventually, they start getting tired. So, the next person has to get up to speed in her lane, stick a hand back, and pull their teammate through the passing zone. That's why a runner's splits are always faster in a relay than they are in an open 400-meter dash. You're always looking forward, and you have somebody to pull you through to the end, which is also somebody else's beginning. You can't let them or the team down, so you push to your limits and beyond.

OKAY, LET'S TALK ABOUT THE RELAY of your life.

You explode out of the blocks as a kid, learn to walk, to run, and to drive away from home and start out on your own. But maybe then your stride falters a bit, and you start looking for direction. Where's the next passing zone? What's going to allow you get back up to speed again, making serious progress? Faced with that challenge, you need to be able to keep your head up, lengthen your stride, deal with the pain, and let the future pull *you* through the end of your split.

Of course, you're passing that baton to yourself, so make sure your momentum is strong! Make the time count!

Every time you get ready to receive the baton, you're looking back at that person who was starting to get weak. And that weakness is actually pushing the next you along, because you're looking back and shouting, "Bring it! We can do this! I'll carry it from here!"

You receive that baton, and then, once you get to that next place, you realize: I was able to pull that exhausted person through, but she got me where I am now. She was pushing *me* to succeed!

You owe a debt to your past self for handing off and putting you in a position to succeed, and you also have a responsibility to your future self to finish as strong as you possibly can to give her momentum.

Don't drop the baton. Deliver it!

CHAPTER FIVE

COMING OUT (NOT *THAT* WAY . . . YET)

M irror therapy—like the kind that helped me in track—doesn't work for everybody.

A lot of people look in the glass and see only what they want to see. Weirdly, that image usually is made up only of the negatives.

The majority—count Shaun T in here—focus on their flaws, not their beauty. A lot of people see their entire histories up to that moment, and they hate themselves for it. (When I look, I still see the chubby round face I had when I weighed 230 pounds. Not fair to current-day me, but true nonetheless.)

I hear it all the time from people who've lost a lot of weight. How they can't stand looking at the photo of themselves at the wedding—the one that forced them to turn the corner. But you have to love that person. That person is the one who got you where you are today! (Hey, round-faced Shaun! You the man!)

I've heard people say: "Oh my God. I don't want to go back

to who I used to be." They tell me how much they hate their "weakness." Sometimes, this is the context of that time they went to a restaurant, had a couple of glasses of wine, lost self-control, and ordered a slice of cheesecake, and said, yes, they wanted it à la mode. Then, when it came, they ate every bite and licked the plate.

Doesn't that sound *good*?

I hate to hear when somebody tells me that story, and makes it clear that they can't forgive themselves for it.

My response is, "You lost 100 pounds. One meal cannot control who you are. And, anyway, you can't reject who you were in that photo, eating those desserts, with all that weight. Because that's the person who helped you reach where you are today.

"So," I'll tell them, "enjoy that cheesecake and the ice cream, and add some extra caramel sauce to it. You have the power to overcome these things, and you can do it no matter what you had for dessert last night."

Love the person you were, even if she broke the scale and struggled to get up off the couch. Because she will eventually stand up, and that's the heroic moment—when you believe in yourself and muster the trust in your future to change direction of your journey.

TRUTHBOMB: Crossing the starting line, where nobody's cheering for you, and nobody believes in you, is always a bigger deal than crossing the finish line, where everybody cheers you on.

It's what you do all by yourself that really counts. That's your power source, and nobody can take that power away from you. *Because it comes from within.*

ONCE I CROSSED MY PERSONAL STARTING line, at age 14, I was in a flat-out sprint. I was busy with choir and schoolwork during the day, and then I'd report to sports practice until dinnertime. When I stepped off the late-bus at 5:10, my grandparents would literally be sitting at the dinner table with a meal laid out and on the table and a kind word for me.

Then, let us pray: "Dear Lord, thank you for this food. . . ."

Dear Lord, I'd think, thank you for Mom-Mom and Pop-Pop. . . .

After dinner, I'd race through my homework and then head off to my night job—usually fast-food related—from 7:00 to 10:00. No room in that schedule for teenage Shaun to get in trouble.

I was a sprinter on the track, but a distance runner with all the activities that packed the rest of my day. And when you're 17, what do you have more of than energy? Better to expend it and make a little pocket money than get in trouble with all the kids who had less Pop-Pop and more free time.

My time was expensive from the get-go, because, even at age 16, I ran my mouth for a living. My first job was as a telemarketer.

Perfect, right?

I pulled on my headset and called random strangers trying to sell them dental insurance. One after another, I interrupted people's dinners, TV watching, and, from the sound of it, their sex lives, as I invaded their homes and tried to sell them something they had never heard of and certainly didn't want to buy from a teenager reading a script. My most frequent response was "click." Alternately, I got lots of "go f&*k yourself!" and "why are you such a dick?"

"Just doing my job, sir," I'd say.

On to my next victim.

It certainly helped me learn to deal with rejection!

If I interrupted you or a family member during your dinner

back then, I apologize. I was never guilty of actually selling any dental insurance. I had way too much sympathy for the people I was interrupting, so I never pressed the matter to meet my quota.

Teenage Shaun was relieved when they fired his ass from that telemarketing job.

On to McDonald's, peddling the kind of food I only rarely eat myself, now. Not that I'm dissing the odd Quarter-Pounder, if you're in a pinch. Twenty-four grams of protein, yo. And it provided me a way to give back to Mom-Mom and Pop-Pop. I'd return home at 10:00 p.m. with a bag of goodies, and we'd all sit down and eat a second dinner. Praise the Lord, and pass the ketchup.

From McD's, it was on to my very best fast-food job, at Chuck E. Cheese's. It was a really big deal back then: Cheap pies and soda, expensive video games, deafening noise, and always, a sweaty human in a rodent costume to provide the entertainment.

I started out as the table-clearer and trash-mover, but one night, when I reported for work, the manager said: "You're Chuck E. tonight."

My first time as a headliner!

I hated putting on the clammy costume—they never really dry out from performance to performance—but once I was inside, I'd give it 100 percent. This was a lesson I'd apply later in my fitness classes: It wasn't about me dressing up as a mouse. I went with the requirements of the moment. To entertain. To bring the energy. To focus on the job at hand, rather than the stink of the Chuck E. costume. When I got lost in a job, there was no room for self-pity. I was *in it*, which meant I was going to *win it*.

The kids deserved that—even the ones who directed well-placed fists at Chuck E.'s most vulnerable regions. I was the entertainment, so I was determined to entertain. And it worked out better for me, too, because I was in a feedback loop: If I was high-energy, the kids responded in kind, which transformed me into a super-rodent. What's more, I found out that I was *good* at it.

TRUTHBOMB: Nothing helps you as much as deciding that, wherever you may be, you're going to take absolutely everything from the experience. Even if you're inside a mouse costume.

When you think of it, this was my first professional dance gig. Once every hour or so, an announcement would come over the intercom asking the kids, "Are you ready for Chuck E. Che-e-e-e-e-e-e-e-ese?"

A shriek went up. Yup. They're ready.

Showtime!

I'd gyrate out onto the stage, full of Chuck E. energy, and start interacting with all of these mechanical creatures on stage while the music blared. I know it's funny to think of your boy Shaun as a giant mouse, but it gave me a taste for the performing life that I still haven't lost. And my audience loved it! Can't ask for more than that: A popular role in a long-running musical in front of an audience hopped up on fountain drinks and pepperoni pizza.

No matter what's going on during my day job now, it couldn't be more difficult than dancing in a mouse suit. Think about that the next time you start hurting at your own job. The fact is, though, that I kind of miss it sometimes. Even a rock-bottom job can take you outside yourself, hook you up with people you'd never meet any other way, and give you skills that just might be useful when you get into your career sweet spot. There's more in common between dancing as Chuck E. Cheese for 20 teenagers and leading an *INSANITY* workout for a thousand people than you might think! I'd love to go back and be Chuck E. for a day. (Yo, Chuck E. corporate, what do you say? Just dry-clean the costume for me, okay?)

Even though the kids treated me like a Looney Tunes character at times, they were also looking for something important from me: An escape, a fantasy sprung to life, a release for the soda-energy throbbing in their veins. It wasn't a dead-end job for a teenager. It was career prep for a guy who would one day need to connect with an amped-up crowd! Without a mouse suit!

What's the equivalent in your life? Maybe not working at a pizza joint. But I'm a big believer in a) doing something really difficult, while b) flooding your brain with positive thoughts. It's possible to break the thought patterns of fear or discouragement, frustration or even embarrassment—all you need to do is find something that makes you feel good that you can use to shout down those negative feelings.

Can you move yourself into a positive groove during minute 22 of an *INSANITY Max 30* workout?

Can you sign up for the half-marathon a half-year from now, even before you've begun your training, and talk yourself straight through to the finish line?

Can you pull some music into the attic next weekend and provide a soundtrack to the hard work of clearing space of stuff you don't need anymore, but somebody else might?

Challenge your body and your ego, and let positive voices and feelings carry you over the starting line. You'll show those muscles who's boss, and you won't believe how good it feels to achieve something you didn't know you could do.

BY HIGH SCHOOL, I ALREADY FELT like I had conquered some pretty enormous challenges. I had taken control of my life, and I was constantly testing myself to see how far I could go and how much I could achieve.

But I wasn't done with difficult challenges, and the biggest one of that time was coming to terms with my sexual identity.

Figuring it out, I went to my usual process. Look myself in the eye, in the mirror, be honest, and figure it out.

I could see that, for the early part of my life, most of my major crushes were on boys, and on my favorite male teachers. I had plenty of friends who were girls, and I was developing into a major jock, as I've said. But my fascination for other boys went beyond a need for friends. It was the dawning of an emotional preference that would grow into a yearning for a physical connection.

And that would lead me back in front of the mirror, where I could be most honest with myself. No arm-pumping sprints this time. Now I was looking myself in the eye and saying, "Okay, you've kissed girls, and done other things with girls that Mom-Mom and Pop-Pop wouldn't approve of. But be honest: Did you really enjoy that?"

Pondering.

"Am I gay?"

More pondering.

Major thought process.

Major look into my soul. Answer: Yes.

It certainly would have been easier *not* to be gay. These were the days before the Supremes (the court, not the girl group) declared marriage equality the law of the land. Before that even seemed possible. The barriers were still huge, and I had to face them and my own truth at the same time.

A LOT OF YOU HAVE HEARD me say: "When the pain begins, that's when the workout begins, and that's when your progress begins." Failure is painful, but it's just another step on your journey unless you let it stop you.

So, back to the mirror.

Wipe the glass clear, maintain eye contact, and be honest about whatever you can't accept about yourself. Then, gather all your best qualities around you, and say, "I'm powerful, I'm happy, I'm good to people, AND I'm _____."

Fill in that blank however you need to.

When I filled the blank in with "gay," so much fell into place for me. It was another big hurdle: acceptance of who I am. And, even though I wasn't ready to shout it into the streets—you didn't do that in 1994—I was at least ready to admit it to myself.

Do you need to schedule a talk with the mirror? If you have to ask, the answer is probably yes. But that should be an exhilarating feeling. What you see when you look in the mirror this time might not be what you expected. It might be scary. But you have more power than anyone else. Know why? Only you live inside your skin, and that's where personal power starts.

You have that.

What will you use it for?

SELF-TEST:
WHERE DID YOU COME FROM?

Now it starts, the superpower self-tests. You'll need to take some time with this. It's when the reading stops and the action begins. Transformation means moving from one way of living to a whole new one, and that requires planning, commitment, and sweat. You've been sitting and reading until now. It's time to work for change in your life.

Let's start with a mirror exercise. Yes, I've spent a lot of time in front of the glass, to examine my warts and blemishes. I also use it as a kind of rearview mirror on my life, so I can check out how the past is influencing my today and my tomorrow. In the first exercise in this book, I'm going to encourage you to do the same. Trust and believe: You won't be able to make any progress on your future unless you've fully examined your past, and then act on that knowledge.

You carry that history in a lot of different ways: It could be the crick in your neck because of the way you sit at your desk, or the plaque in your heart because of your dietary habits. It could be the friends who stick with you through thick and thin, or the ones who stick to you like leeches. It could be the regrets and resentments that tie you up emotionally, so you're not free to live and love the way you'd like.

Let's invest some time in a backward glance to better wipe your mirror clear and see yourself as you really are today.

EXERCISE #1

Get a check-up. Your body is a walking, talking historical record of everything you've been through, and the most common causes of death are tied to long-term health habits. If your stresses are tied to your personal history—and whose aren't?—you need to dig them up and deal. As your doctor examines your health history, she'll also be helping you write and rectify the most troubling elements of your past. *If you help her to do so.* So, be honest with her, and yourself.

ACTION PLAN: Work with your doctor to develop three concrete steps you'll take. For instance: 1. Lose ten pounds, 2. Commit to a sleep schedule, 3. Limit drinking to weekends and even then only one or two glasses. And schedule another appointment to check your progress.

EXERCISE #2

Do a fitness test. I threw a killer test at the beginning of my *INSANITY* workout, which might have scared off as many people as it lured into that program. But I did it for a reason: To know where you're going, you need to know where you are and have a benchmark to help measure your progress. I'm not going to suggest you go there, unless you're already at a pretty high level of fitness. But, if you've laid off for a while, try these five simple fitness tests.

1. Go out to the track at the high school, and see how far you can walk or run in 15 minutes.

2. Get down in a plank position—elbows under your shoulders, spine and legs in a straight line, ankles bent at 90 degrees, toes on the floor—and see how long you can hold it.

3. How many push-ups can you do in a minute?

4. How many crunches can you do in a minute?

5. Sit on the floor. Can you move to a standing position without using your hands?

Make a note of your results. If there will be a physical component to your transformation plan, it'll be helpful (and encouraging!) to see just how far you come.

ACTION PLAN: Once you have your fitness baseline, schedule time to really work on improving your numbers. Will this take a commitment? Of course. Why did you buy this book?

EXERCISE #3

Review the relationships. Pull out the photo boxes in mom's attic (and in your Facebook history). This won't be a simple stroll down memory lane. Instead, use the photo record to really think about the relationships in your life. Distant or absent father? Bullying older siblings? Were you a loner? Were you always howling or unhappy as a 3-year-old? Did you hate that sweater your mom made you wear in junior high? Did you have Mom-Mom and Pop-Pop figures who unfailingly brought the love? What made you happiest? When was your best age? And your worst (*aside* from middle school, that is)? Catalog it all, positive and negative. Think about what made those high-light moments so great, and what about the negative times was so painful. Consider how you're carrying those hurts and helpers into your current world.

ACTION PLAN: At the end of Chapter Eight I'll give you complete instructions on gauging the strength of your inner circle. If this chapter's exercise hurts, you might need to skip ahead to do that one now. It's *that* important.

EXERCISE #4

Review the disasters. This will hurt. That's why you need to do it, of course. And as you go through the pain of each of them, ask yourself: Have I recovered, or am I still suffering from . . . my parents' divorce, my dad's death, when I moved across the country during sixth grade. Whatever it was that hurt you most, heal from it, however you need to do that. If you don't, it might hold you back for the rest of your life.

ACTION PLAN: There's only so much guidance I can offer here. It took me six years and two counselors to work through the aftermath of sexual abuse. The more painful this disaster inventory is for you, the more you need to reach for help. Ask friends for referrals on counselors; they're getting help, and you may need it too.

EXERCISE #5

Search out the shame. As an abuse survivor, I know all about shame. I was attacked sexually by an adult, bullied into silence, and made to feel that, somehow, it was all my fault. Shame punishes you for being who you are, not for what you've done. So, it goes to the very core of your identity. Can you see why it's so important to deal with it? A counselor can help; that's how I got past mine.

ACTION PLAN: Some of these tips and strategies come from a psychiatrist, in fact: Harold H. Bloomfield, MD, shared them with *Prevention* magazine, and I adapted them here. Check out his book *Making Peace with Your Past* for more ways to heal your personal history.

EXERCISE #6

Release the resentment. Compile a list of the people who held you back, who didn't believe in you, who actively tried to sabotage you. Consider why you let them block you, how they exerted their power, how their influence still affects you today. Print those letters out. Write names on envelopes, and stick the letters in them. And then . . . this is important . . . destroy them. Whether you burn them, flush them, rip them into a million pieces and throw them in different trash cans, savor watching those sentiments get completely dismantled and destroyed. Then, put the resentments—however justified—entirely behind you. It takes precious energy to keep resentments alive, and they trap you in the worst moments of your past. They aren't worth it. Send their dirty deeds up in smoke, and never look back.

ACTION PLAN: Open a file on your computer and write letters to the people who hurt you the most.

EXERCISE #7

Let go of regrets. I'm totally with fellow Jersey guy Frank Sinatra, who sang "regrets, I've had a few. . . ." But, if you cultivate those in your emotional garden, they can kill every other flower in there. So, forgive yourself for the ones you had a hand in, dismiss the ones others inflicted on you, and then give them up. As my father-in-law, Bill Blokker, says, your windshield should be bigger than your rearview mirror. To keep an eye on the road ahead, with all of its twists, turns, off-ramps, and opportunities, you need to stop regretting the turns you missed or the crashes you suffered. That's behind you now.

ACTION PLAN: Take the time to explore each of your major regrets, understand why they hurt so much, and harvest any lessons you can from what happened. Then use your mental discipline to keep your focus forward from now on. Shrink the rearview, expand your windshield. Now *drive*.

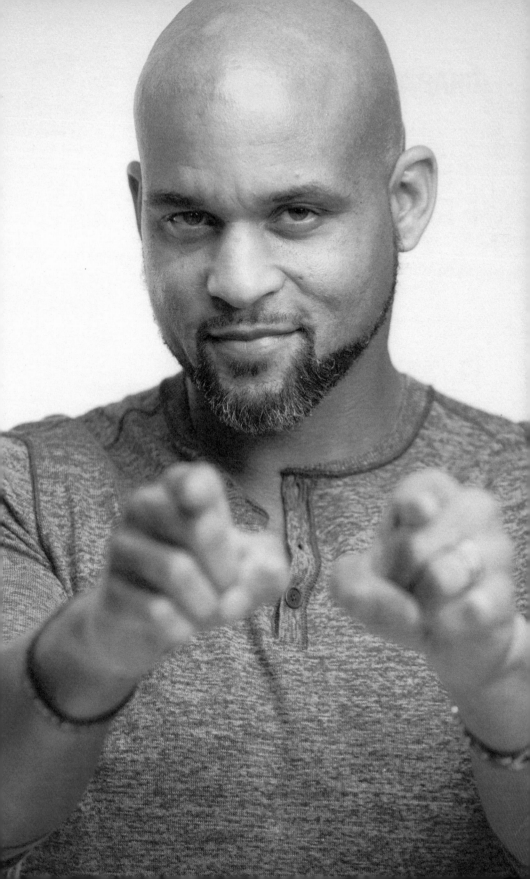

CHAPTER SIX

THE FRESHMAN 50

Picture a long hallway, lined with doors.

You're walking along, considering them. Light is escaping out from underneath them, and you can hear sounds coming from within.

Behind one, you can hear a party. People are having a great time. But you don't know any of these people, and besides, nobody invited you.

Behind another, you can hear a business meeting going on, and people are accomplishing great things. But the conversation is over your head, and you strain to make sense of it.

Behind yet another, you hear a mom, dad, and a couple of kids—and they're enjoying the kind of chaos you get when a family goes nuclear. But it's not your family.

At the final door, you hear a group workout. There's a teacher calling out exercises and motivating people—*"Come on, y'all! Dig deeper!"*—and it sounds exciting, but it's probably too hard for you.

You're not alone in the hallway. There are others who have been shut out of those rooms, as well. And when they're not trying to sneak in through a keyhole or slide under the door, they're looking around to clear the crowd from the hallway, and they do that by hating on everybody within earshot.

You just toured a hallway I'm still walking down myself, every day of my life. But why? I'm authentically shy at heart. What you see is TV Shaun T; Little Shauny is still holding on to mom's leg not wanting to go to preschool.

Will I be accepted if I knock for entry? Can I handle the relationships, the work, the challenge? And who's that loud-mouth workout leader, anyway? (Trust and believe: Even real-life Shaun T is intimidated by DVD Shaun T, sometimes.)

The chapter ahead is all about the doors I pushed through over the course of my life. I didn't feel good approaching any of them, but I wanted to be inside. So, I took a deep breath and entered, even when I didn't think that I belonged. And that has made all the difference in my life.

So, while you're reading about my "doors," I want you to be thinking about your own hallway. What doors are you pressing your ear against but aren't pushing through? As you read my story, I want you to think about knocking on a few of those scary doors yourself.

THE FIRST DOORWAY I WANT YOU to consider is the one to the kitchen of my mom's house in Deptford. It's the middle of the night, so the refrigerator is humming quietly. And all of the kitchen cabinets are closed.

But Shaun is always hungry. That's why he used to stuff Wonder Bread into his underwear.

You read that right.

I didn't starve at my house, growing up. But our pantry wasn't exactly bursting with after-school snacks, either. My mom pulled it together for breakfast and dinner, and I got a free lunch at school because my family was on government assistance. So, I was on an economic diet: I could only eat what we could afford, which wasn't an ounce more than we actually needed.

There was no snack time after we pushed back from the dinner table at 7:30 p.m. Even when Ennis and I were going through our growth spurts, we'd be powerfully hungry. But there just wasn't an answer to "Mom, I'm hungry!" once dinner was over.

That's when my kitchen raids started.

I had a brilliant strategy.

The house grew quiet after bedtime, but my belly wouldn't shut up, so I would sneak out of my bedroom, barely touch the stairs so they wouldn't creak, tiptoe into the kitchen, then jump up on the counter. No wonder I was such a good hurdler in high school.

My mom knew to store the bread on a high shelf, to keep it away from Ennis and me. Not high *enough*, Mom!

Standing on the counter, I'd stretch for that blue, red, and yellow spotted bag, then open it *so carefully*. For a little kid sneaking around in the middle of the night, that crinkly sound was like a foghorn that was going to wake the whole neighborhood. My salivary glands would be jetting as I'd reach in the bag for a slice or two—only enough so nobody would notice what was missing. Then came the really crafty part: I'd mash and fold the bread up into a little, fragrant dough ball. Wonder was great that way!

Then, I'd drop the dough ball into my underwear.

Why not just eat the damn bread right then and there, you ask?

Too risky!

If I'd ever been caught "bread-handed" in the kitchen, or on the stairs, the game would be over. Wonder in the lockbox, next time. But, with the bread ball safely stowed in my underwear, I could claim that I was just getting a glass of water—the only no-limit sustenance we had when I was a kid.

After I stashed my slice(s), I'd reverse the process— off-counter with a Spiderman jump, tiptoe across the cold kitchen floor, creak-free sneak up the stairs, and then back into bed, heart pounding. At last: Time for the midnight Wonder snack. Builds strong bodies in 12 ways!

(Note to modern bread-eaters: The reason that the Wonder doughball formed so nicely? It was the gluten! Now, imagine *that* clogging up your digestive tract.)

Even when I moved over to my grandparents' house, where Mom-Mom wasn't exactly holding back rations, we weren't snacking 24/7. The pastor and his missus believed in keeping *all* appetites under control.

So, when I went away to college, I wasn't ready for all the freedoms that I suddenly had.

Now, let's back up a minute. I was a track athlete in high school. Colleges offered me scholarships to run around in circles for their glory. But, my mom made the right call: "You need a scholarship that's going to work your mind," she told me, "so you don't have to focus on your body and run."

Well, yeah.

So, my choice was pretty obvious: I'd accept a fistful of academic grants from Rowan University and concentrate on my studies.

Some of you who are reading this are on your own weight-loss journey. At this point in my story, I took a big fat wrong turn. One of the common mistakes people make is thinking that the metabolic machine they are as a teenager will keep on firing as they move into their late twenties and thirties. By the time they realize that it shut down—the decline starts at around age 25, people!—they may already be 20 or 30 pounds past their ideal weight.

It's another way we'll never be who we were in high school, when our bodies were pumping out human growth hormone (HGH), and we were funneling those cheeseburger calories into repeated growth spurts. But as you age, and your metabolism declines and the HGH jets stop firing, you need to make adjustments to your diet (less) and exercise (more). This isn't anybody's fault: It's how we're built. But ignoring it won't make it go away, okay?

Back in college, I was an expert at ignoring a small problem until it became a big problem. I was shocked at freshman orientation at Rowan, when they handed me my meal card. My scholarship was for room, board, and tuition, and I made the most of all three. I did fine in my classes, but I could hardly wrap my brain around the concept of unlimited free food. I quickly wrapped my hand around a fork, and didn't hesitate to use it.

This food card is *full*!

Soon I was stuffed, too.

I quickly caught onto the fact that my meal card worked in the cafeteria *and off campus*. I could order Domino's pizza whenever I wanted to. And I always wanted to, even after midnight. Much more convenient than pulling a dough ball out of my tighty-whities. I was Chuck E. Cheese all over again, but instead of playing an overstuffed mouse, I *became* one.

And, because I was now focused on academics instead of athletics, I wasn't balancing the calorie intake with afterburners during track practice.

As I ate my way through freshman year, I became aware that my body was changing. I elevated through several changeovers in the waist size of my jeans, rationalizing that it was a style thing. And, in the beginning, I was blind to what was actually happening to me.

Remember how I hid in my closet as a little kid? Now, my dorm room served the same function. The bigger I got, the less I showed my round face around campus. The Shaun who loved to dance at high-school parties was replaced by the Shaun who holed up in the dorm after class. I was a communications major who became increasingly shy of public places.

It wasn't long before I became completely stressed about how I looked, and that was on top of the usual stuff that's bugging your average 19-year-old. I was coming to terms with everything from my sexuality (not hetero) to whether or not I was going to become president of the United States (not yet).

It was a lot to handle.

When I boss y'all around on *INSANITY* and *FOCUS T25®* and tell you to dig deeper, I know what that means, personally. I had to climb up from a deep layer of fat myself. I know what it feels like to feel uncomfortable with how you look and to have clothes in the closet that don't fit anymore, and I'm still connected to that part of my journey every day. So, I can tap into your journey, too, if that's what you've experienced.

My weight gain wasn't just about easy access to a meal card.

I was swiping hard for another reason, aside from how good pizza tastes.

In high school, I wanted to be accepted like everyone else. Who doesn't want to be accepted? I knew I was gay, but I still did my best to convince myself and others that I liked girls. If I was good at being Chuck E. Cheese, hell, I could also fake heterosexuality, I guess.

But in offering that crucial lie to the world, I opened the door to my weight gain as well.

TRUTHBOMB: If you define yourself by a negative, that negative spreads to other areas of your life.

My "problem" when I got to college: Girls thought I was "cute." Even roly-poly me.

And why not? I was a nice guy, kind to people, plenty of friends. But, because I wasn't owning my sexuality publicly yet, I was being hit on by women.

It's a strange thing to complain about, but it was stressful for me. I couldn't respond, and I couldn't explain it to them.

That made me seem stuck-up, when I was actually just stuck in my closet again. I was okay with my status as a gay man myself, but I wasn't ready for that to be my public profile.

My response to that tension back then: I ate and ate and ate. I realize now that, on some level, my reasoning was: If I blimped out, maybe women would stop hitting on me.

It's not an unusual reason for weight gain, in fact. Sexuality is a huge issue, no matter who you want to date. People can be afraid of intimacy, or undecided on preference. Maybe they don't want to be in that game at all. So, they put themselves on the sideline by making choices that make them ugly in their own eyes. It's a really good excuse for not playing the dating game at all.

That was my strategy: I tried to eat myself out of romance with the women I was rejecting.

At the beginning of my sophomore year, I was overdue for a mirror moment. It came one morning as I stepped out of the shower and spotted an incredible hulk through the fog.

Whoa! Is that all *me*?

Wipe the glass clean. Yup, all me.

I literally said, out loud, "Oh my God. This is horrible!"

I don't know if anybody heard me say it, but it was loud enough to wake *me* up.

My formerly slim, athletic self—I weighed 178 the day of my high-school graduation—had been transformed. I looked into the glass and suddenly saw exactly what I had become—50 pounds' worth of uncomfortable in my own skin.

We all have imperfections that we don't like about ourselves. For me, it's my face. And, it's not because of how I look now, it's because I remember how big and round my face became when I gained weight. It's like every slice of pizza went there to live, and my face assumed the shape of an extra-large with cheese.

One reason why I work out as hard as I do right now is because I remember, painfully, how my face looked in the mirror that day. But, when I think of that image, it's not the physical appearance that I remember disliking so much.

We all have something that we don't like about ourselves; that's the reason why many of us exercise, or choose the clothes we do, or put on makeup and color our hair.

It's not the thing, it's the *thing*.

Let me explain.

My weight, at 228 pounds, wasn't the right thing for me, but that wasn't really what was out of kilter. It was my balance in life, and my weight was a physical manifestation of the disconnect I was living between the man that I was pretending to be and the man that I really was.

I have a photo of myself that I took when I weighed 224 pounds, down 4 pounds from my maximum weight. You might not recognize me at that size, but here's what I see: The guy who helped me reach where I am today. I reached that weight when I had only just begun my weight-loss journey, but I was already feeling so much better than I had at my max. I made the crucial connection between how much I'd lost and how much better I felt. And, I'm being honest when I tell you that, if I had felt good at 224, I could have stopped right there and been fine with it. But Shaun at 224 was not living the kind of life that I wanted to be living, and that's the realization that began to change everything.

TRUTHBOMB: It's not about the weight. It's about feeling your best and being happy—however you define that.

If 20-year-old Shaun felt good at 224 pounds—physically and emotionally—and sustained that feeling, he would have gone on to another career. And it wouldn't make one bit of difference if I'd chosen another life, and that weight, *as long as it was my choice*.

But, I had a different goal in mind, and it sprang directly from my weight gain.

The first step on that new road took me across the campus. I took a deep breath and pushed through the door to the gym. I didn't feel I belonged there anymore—certainly not looking the way I did. But I went ahead, found an open treadmill, and ran as hard as I could. Ten minutes was about all this former track star could manage in the beginning.

Watch my DVDs, and you'll hear me say, "Go for as long as you can, and then stop. Any activity is better than none. Just do better tomorrow." And that's me speaking to you, but also to my 20-year-old self, to encourage him as well.

It was exhausting for me back then. Uncomfortable. But, I knew how great I felt that first time that Coach Anderson showed me what it felt like to tap into my reserve strength. I knew that I liked that feeling, and I felt, deep down, that pushing myself through the discomfort on the treadmill was what I needed to do. I just wanted to weigh less than 220 pounds!

Every day after my mirror moment, I opened the door to my future by going to the gym to pound the treadmill. That's all I had the confidence for. I could see the fit guys working in the weight room, but they had abs and biceps, so obviously they knew what the hell they were doing.

I did not have those muscles or know those secrets, and I knew I needed to take my time building up my physical strength, along with my confidence.

I always started my workout with the same 10-minute run. That was my foundation to spring up from. What's yours?

Word to the gym-shy: Remember that even the muscular guys—maybe especially the muscular guys—were beginners at one time. The fitter they are, the more they're bouncing back from something themselves. And maybe that something is similar to what you've gone through. Give them a chance to help you. Give yourself a chance to *be* helped. The smart ones will admire what you're doing, because they remember how difficult it was for them, too.

People often tell me that they can't go to the gym because they feel out of place. They look at me and say "Well, you've never been through this. You don't know how it feels."

And, I say to them "Yes, I have."

I remember exactly how it felt on the first day that I walked up to the weight-room door, took a breath, and said, "I need to add this to my journey."

I still didn't have a real fitness plan or any understanding of physiology, but after a few weeks of running the treadmill, at least I felt the motivation to try. That in itself was a fitness breakthrough.

In the weight room, I was in full faking-it mode, looking at people out of the corner of my eye and trying to imitate what they were doing. But, mostly, I was just hoping nobody would notice me!

Think of that if you're ever in a hotel conference room with a thousand other people at a *Shaun T Live* event. If you have to fake it until you make it that day, you have something in common with the guy in the front of the room barking instructions at you on the 20-foot-tall TV screen. We'll get through this together, you hear?

In fact, it didn't matter what I did on the treadmill or in the weight room, early on. I was lucky enough to avoid injury, and whatever I was doing helped me hit 219 pounds, my first goal.

I'm talking about a 9-pound weight loss here, but it might as well have been 90 pounds. I felt amazing!

Please, please, believe me when I tell you that the numbers are always relative and individual.

> **TRUTHBOMB:** Whatever defines progress for you and makes you feel better, you have to take a moment and congratulate yourself. Enjoy the benefit. Lock the memory of that great feeling into place, even if you feel you still have 40 more pounds to lose. It's the feeling that matters most, not the number. And all that matters is what *you're* feeling, not anybody else. Own that!

YOU MAY THINK THAT MY FOOD challenges are over. Shaun T is a dietary deity, right?

Not hardly.

At the end of the calendar year, I like to clear my schedule, take a week off, find a swimming pool and a lounge chair, and kick it for a week.

Actually, it usually works out to just 5 days, because who has the time? But, when I'm on vacation, my diet takes a vacation, too.

So, picture your man, Shaun T, who coaches people through 5-, 10-, 30-, 50-pound weight losses, doing absolutely nothing and eating absolutely everything for 5 straight days.

It feels just as good for me as it would for you.

Now, I like to set a good example, even when it comes to setting a good example of how selectively bad Shaun T can be. None of us is perfect, but especially not me on vacation.

Here's the deal, though: I understand both the importance of fueling my body for the life I want to live and cutting loose every now and then, so I don't drive myself crazy. The real danger in your diet isn't the occasional fun food, it's that you'll use that single jelly doughnut you ate as a sign that you're hopeless, and then finish off the full dozen.

Don't fall off the wagon and stay down there in the muck. Instead, plan your leaps, enjoy them, and then go back to the kinds of foods that will do the very best job of fueling your exercise plan and maintaining your body for the long run. Most of the time, I live on sweet potatoes, bananas, lean meats, water, and fruit. And, the servers in the restaurants near my home in Arizona know I'm going to customize their menus for maximum nutrition.

But, that's not all I'm about, food-wise.

You'll see at the end of this chapter that I'm all about eating 85-percent healthy and 15-percent fun. Stick with that, and you'll move from thick to thin, I guarantee it.

My grandfather used to tell me that my body was my temple. Right, Pop-Pop. But a temple can get kind of boring, so I invite in the fun foods to keep the party going. That's fine every now and then, so long as I remember that I also need to clean up after the party. There's a balance to everything I do and everything I eat; it's the key to success for everybody.

We're all vulnerable to foods that will make us feel lousy if we eat too much of them. And, that's just what the food manufacturers have in mind as they sneak sweet and salty flavors, plus fat and sugar overloads, into snacks and entrées so we won't be able to quit eating them. Your body has craved those energy-packed foods since prehistory, because they helped your apelike ancestors survive in the bush.

But, we don't live in the bush anymore. We live in Candyland. So, our eating instincts aren't serving us well. They're overserving us, in fact. And, in many cases, that's because we use food for many more things than just nourishment. Our relationships with food are all mixed up with control, with comfort, and with how we socialize and relate to the people around us. Food can have a dramatic psychological hold, and when we're not in a good head-space, one of the first things that tends to happen is that our eating habits veer off-track. That's why I like to give myself permission to cut loose when

I'm on vacation—I know that's a setting where I'm already going to be relaxed and feeling good, so I'm not going to be driven to the buffet table by anything other than hunger.

I want you to encourage yourself to take some time to have your mirror moment when it comes to your relationship with food. Set aside the excuses and the reasoning and understand the difference between the thing (a surface difficulty that annoys you) and The Thing (the underlying reason for it).

Example:

> **The thing:** needing a glass or three of wine to unwind in the evening.
>
> **THE THING:** the life stressors behind that "need."
>
>
> **The thing:** eating from the ice cream carton, rather than a nice little bowl.
>
> **THE THING:** how your mom used food as a reward and as a punishment when you were a kid.

See what I'm saying? You need to separate the behavior from the cause, the thing from The Thing.

And once you've done that, can you accept and appreciate the person who does what she does for a reason? Sometimes, a very complex reason that will take time to sort out?

I hope so.

No matter where you are in your journey, you owe yourself at least that much, especially if you've been dissing yourself for all you aren't. Here's what you *are*: A person in progress.

That's why I urge you to look hard at any past version of yourself that you previously rejected, or turned away from, ashamed. Until you accept that person, and give thanks for that step on the pathway to now, you'll have a barrier that will keep you from your heart's desire.

If you accept that person back then, you can thrive now.

The same negative thing that defined you in the past, whether it was a weight gain or fear of public speaking or a bad relationship or a drug problem, can provide the energy to push you forward into a better new life. It's time to stop denying your former self and learn how to understand who you were, and love that person, and congratulate that person, and find your way forward using the head start that earlier version of you provided.

Look fear in the eye, take control of your emotions, and you will *live* the life you deserve and were destined to live.

SELF-TEST:
IS IT THE THING, OR *THE THING?*

Earlier in this chapter I was distinguishing between small-scale behaviors and the big issues they spring from. Below, you'll find five common unhealthy behaviors, equally common motivators for them, and solutions that stop the behaviors by answering the motivator in a healthy way. Once you get the hang of it, you can play along with your own "things," understand The Things that might cause them, and come up with your own solutions. (Plus, as a bonus, I'll give you my Shaun T's Five Rules of Food, which for many of us is the ultimate thing, and The Thing.)

the thing: your soda addiction

THE THING: energy ebbs and flows during the day

Solution: It's a fairly complicated subject, so I don't want to oversimplify, but I'd advise you to start looking at the causes for energy crashes. It could be that you're undervaluing sleep and overvaluing Facebook, *Jimmy Fallon*, or other late-night distractions. Or, it could be that you simply crave the caffeine in your soda of choice and could get your fix from low- or no-calorie tea or coffee instead. Or, it could be that your taste for sweet carbs is leading to a big energy crash later in the day. Or, it could be all of those things. But your soda addiction is trying to tell you something. Are you listening?

the thing: texting while driving

THE THING: your need for social connection

Solution: You know you can shut off those notifications, right? And that a silent phone is better than a dead user, right? But, there is an intense reward-feedback system in place with text messages and other phone blips and bleeps: They remind you of the people you love (or simply people you know), and they give your brain a shot of happy juice (the hormone dopamine) every time you plug into them. We all need to connect, so maybe, if you do a better job of scheduling those lunches with friends, those phone calls to your mom, your after-work get-togethers with clients or workmates, you'll feel less desperate to answer every incoming text, when the next one might just kill you or an innocent bystander who wanders into your path.

the thing: those mean comments or passive-aggressive silences you keep flinging at your spouse or kids

THE THING: unexpressed anger over bigger problems in the relationships

Solution: Make a note of when you lash out. Is it over a mess you find on the kitchen counter? Is it when your spouse stays late at the office for the third time that week? Or, when you make an effort over dinner, and nobody says a word? Instead of storing up that anger, find a calm moment and explain your feelings. Your family can't hear what you don't say. Find a time and a way to say it, and seek a solution instead of just throwing attitude around.

the thing: you blew off your workout today

THE THING: your lack of belief in yourself, which leads you to self-sabotage your self-improvement projects

Solution: Engineer some can't-miss successes for yourself. I've seen a lot of people attempt to take U-turns in their lives, and a lot of them are going so fast in the wrong direction that their car flips when they try to make a turn. Don't be like them! So, instead of making huge promises to yourself, make small ones that you know you can keep. If you're stuck on the couch, don't say you're going to run the New York City marathon 4 months from now. Instead, commit to 15 minutes of exercise—any kind—a day. When that becomes easy, bump it up to a half-hour. You want to commit to small changes but honor the commitment. Then, you'll feel more confident about the big changes, and you'll be able to turn the car safely, without a wreck. U-turn, here we come.

the thing: your cupboard is filled with sweet treats, and you just can't help but snack on them

THE THING: your troubled relationship with food, where you swing from bingeing to starving, and don't feel good about either

Solution: Shaun T's 85/15 food plan! The basic principle is this: Eat 85-percent healthy and 15-percent fun. Pretty simple, right? More important, it's *realistic*. Just keep the following five rules in mind, and your body will be a temple . . . *and* you can keep the party going in there, just like I do.

SHAUN T'S
FiVE RULES OF FOOD

RULE #1
What you eat is more important than how much you exercise. I'm not dissing exercise; it's a pillar of my life. But I do want you to pay attention to what you put into your body. Make 85-percent good food choices—the veggies, the whole fruit, the protein—that will keep your calorie counts low, your belly full, and your nutrition up. Add exercise on top of that, and you're on the way to feeling amazeballs every day.

RULE #2
Your eating plan is working if you're a little hungry sometimes. I am not saying "starve yourself." Just find ways to get through your hunger pangs. When I was gaining my freshman 50, I would take the slightest stomach gurgle as a direct order from my belly: "Feed me!" But a hunger pang will only last 10 to 15 minutes, and then go away. And, trust me, if a gurgle hits at 10:00 a.m., throw yourself into that project at work, or call a girlfriend to vent about

your lousy boyfriend. Suffer a 4:00 p.m. craving? Don't give in! Do one of my 5-minute Facebook workouts instead. Or take a walk. You don't even have to change your clothes! Midnight snack attack? I don't think so. Dial up a YouTube video instead. Plus, you save 100 percent of the calories you don't eat, so find ways to get through that hunger pang. I promise you, it will end. Willpower is a muscle you develop by—how else?—exercising it.

RULE #3

It's okay to have fun (15 percent of the time), as long as you climb back up onto the wagon afterward (85 percent of the time). I've never been a big fan of New Year's resolutions. Why not resolve, and follow through, on April 17th, as well? Or any other day, for that matter? Another big problem with resolutions: When people break them on January 23rd, they take it as a sign that they're just no good at working out or eating right, and they abandon their best intentions entirely. So, that's where the 15-percent fun comes through on this food plan. You're going to have your indulgences, and I want you to enjoy them fully, like I do. Just go back to the foods you should be eating 85 percent of the time right after. One Cinnabon isn't going to bust your belt, but being disgusted with yourself, and chasing it with fried chicken for lunch and a chocolate sundae after dinner, just might. Fun foods are temporary, the best foods are a favor that you do for yourself your whole life long. Plan for them accordingly.

RULE #4

Only let the best foods in your grocery cart, your house, and your mouth (85 percent of the time, anyway). It cracks me up, and makes me a little sad, when people point with horror at the junk food their kids eat. Tell me, Mom or Dad, how did that giant bottle of soda, the Costco tray of pastries, that sloppy cheeseburger and fries, get into the cupboard or the fridge or your car window in the first place, and then into a kid's hands? Right, Mom or Dad bought it! Junior ain't driving through the drive-thru, you are! Your grocery cart is a sacred place. Only put the very best foods into it. How do you find those? Shop the edges of the store, where the vegetables, meat, eggs, and dairy (if you can tolerate that) live. The closer your food is to its natural state—straight off the cow, the pig, the chicken, the farm—the better. When food processors start adding ingredients, they're almost always of the trans-fatty, super-salty, and high-fructose variety. Don't go there, for your sake, and for your kids' sake. Remember, *you* are in control!

RULE #5

Losing a pound or two a week is a healthy rate; small losses add up to big ones, and they're sustainable. One of the things that drives me nuts about weight-loss reality-TV shows is that they make such a big deal out of giant weekly weigh-ins. Contestants on those shows might be dropping 5 pounds a week for a shot at the big payday, but they're dooming themselves to putting that weight back on equally quickly. I know the struggles they go through because I hosted one of those shows. If you lose a ton of weight every week, your body goes into panic mode and overrides whatever extreme method you've been using to lose that weight. You're *not* winning that fight. Instead, focus on food and exercise changes that become part of your life for the rest of your life. The weight loss may be slower—a pound a week is a good goal—but it is more likely to be sustainable. That's why I say 85-percent good foods, 15-percent fun. Who can't live with that?

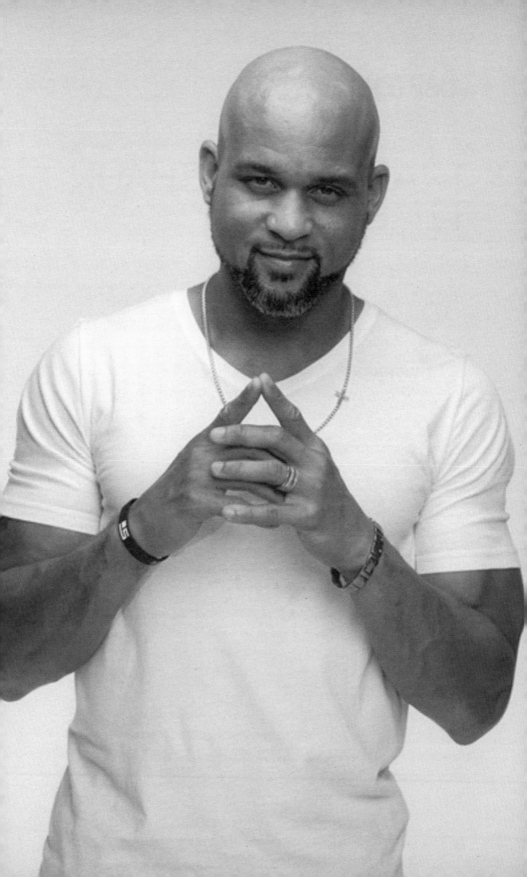

CHAPTER SEVEN

TRANSFORMASHAUN TIME

TRUTHBOMB: Real progress doesn't begin until you step outside of your comfort zone.

True in my workouts.

True in your life, too.

We have all gotten trapped in the wrong kind of comfort zone, when what we're comfortable with is killing us. I wonder if you're in one of those right now?

I wouldn't blame you. The majority of us go along with a lot of stuff simply to keep everybody comfortable.

Stuff like:

Okay, your boss is an incompetent hothead, but if everybody in the office just keeps quiet, a paycheck will arrive on schedule every 2 weeks.

Yes, your sister-in-law makes life hell for the whole family, but if we just avoid certain topics at the Thanksgiving-dinner table, we'll all survive until the pecan pie is served.

Right, your "friend" makes you squirm with the way she competes with you and tears you down and talks behind your back, but you've been together such a long time. It's so much easier to keep seeing her than to watch her go ballistic if you move on.

And, oh my, this overstuffed recliner is so *comfortable*. This afternoon isn't a great time to get up and move.

In all four of these scenarios, the comfortable thing is to keep quiet, avoid confrontation, and keep doing what you're doing.

When you call out the boss, tie a bell on the she-cat sister-in-law, turn your back on your frenemy, or get out of the chair, it's uncomfortable . . . in the beginning.

But, when you push through, you realize that you don't have to deal with any of that "comfortable" bullstuff anymore.

Even better, you prove to yourself that you're strong enough to create a change for the better in your own life. So, what makes *you* uncomfortable? It could be your direct link to a better world. Squirm on over there, why don't you?

SHAUN-MINUS-4-POUNDS WAS SWEATY ON THE TREADMILL, and he didn't feel like he even belonged in the gym. I'd found my *dis*comfort zone alright, but I couldn't believe how good I felt after I lost the first 4 pounds.

It's not much, right? After all, I was still large.

But here's the key: Propelled by the amazeballs feeling of progress, I developed new goals immediately after I'd reached the first one of weighing in at under 220 pounds. I translated the new way I was feeling into a new direction for my life.

I told my best confidante, the mirror, "I'm changing my major from communications to sports science, to health and exercise." If I could get other people to experience the same shift I had, from hopeless to hopeful, to see a result that made me feel better than I had in years, I'd found my life passion.

I didn't know if I could make a living at it; I just knew it would be deeply rewarding to me, so I placed the bet. On me. I enrolled in health and exercise classes and studied kinesiology, exercise physiology, health promotion, and health behavior. I wanted to understand what could carry me beyond my mirror moment, and then help other people feel exactly as good as I did.

You should find healthy habits and exercise opportunities that make you feel great, and then, naturally, you'll want to find more and more of that great feeling, and lock it in for the rest of your life. Shaun T doesn't whip out the "tough-trainer" act too often. I never want to shame *anybody* into doing *anything*. Instead, I want them to taste a little of the joy I felt when I lost my first 4 pounds, and keep the good times rolling in search of more of that joy. I'm all carrot and no stick, and not just because carrots have a lot of fiber and vitamin A. It's because life ought to be a pleasure, and your healthy habits should give you more and more of that.

Keep in mind that there was nothing magic that helped me turn the tide against the 50 pounds I'd gained. My "program" was actually kind of random: no trainer, no diet, no plan in particular. Just a deep desire to change.

> **TRUTHBOMB:** If you look hard in the mirror and begin to see yourself in a new way, you can become that new person.

This wasn't about other people or what they thought of me. *I* wasn't satisfied, *I* didn't feel good. So, *I* took steps toward transformaShaun. The first step in the process was that I knew I needed to change.

The second step was that I trusted that I could make a change, and believed in every step that was taking me there. Before there were any results the rest of the world could see, *I made changes inside*. That was the difference between 228-pound Shaun and the man I was on my way to becoming.

Here's something not a lot of people know. As my studies accelerated, I found my way into . . . square dancing!

Yee haw! Doh-see-doh, Shaun T!

Okay, it wasn't the kind of dance I'd end up doing for a living, but there is a lesson here. The first step on a new road probably won't be the one that delivers you where you want to go. But, a step is a step, and you should treasure all progress, no matter how small—even if it's onto the square dance floor with Clem the Caller, and what you really want is to step in with Lady Gaga at halftime during the Super Bowl!

I can't say I was ever crazy about the allemande left, but I did love translating my physical abilities into the rhythms and patterns of dance.

I'm one of those people who has loved dancing for a long time.

I can remember being at my 8th birthday party, and the music came on, and I was just *in it*. People must have been laughing and paying attention, because I played to that. It gave me a reason to actually enjoy being with people. Maybe they weren't so awful after all?

That same year, I asked my mom if I could be a ballerina.

I used that specific word, too: *ballerina*.

They were so pretty! The outfits! The hairdos! The pink tights!

My mom gave me a look, which is probably why I still remember it today. She said, "I don't think you'd want to do that."

My mom isn't a judgmental person. She was Pop-Pop's daughter, and he was the best example of tolerance: His church accepted every person in his community. So, I know now that she meant her response to be something more along the lines of, "Shaun, a ballerina is a girl dancer, and you aren't a girl."

But, what I heard was: Boys don't dance.

So, imagine my delight when I was flipping around the TV dial a few years later, and came across cheerleading competitions. Okay, lots of girls in short skirts. But, in the middle of them, there was always one dude who was really good at holding up the pyramid or catching an 80-pounder when she flew in for a landing.

I was shocked. I was thrilled! Mom was wrong! Boys can dance! Maybe there was a place for me in this world, after all!

I started to look for opportunities to pull on my dancing shoes and try on a choreographer hat. I was president of the E.R.A.S.E. club in high school—End Racism and Sexism Every-where—and we worked with the drill team to choreograph routines for pep rallies. It was just a lot of stomping and clap-ping, but isn't that how a lot of great things begin? With a lot of noise and fun? I was finally on my way.

Of course, all this was strictly amateur stuff. I didn't get any proper dance training until college. But, it isn't always about the formal training. I had been able to move my ass when the DJ spun at a party. And, between the gym and my classwork, and the dance shows and cheerleader competitions I watched on TV, I was actually training my brain and learn-ing the movements. By doing that, I was starting to build one skill on top of another into a personal superpower that would eventually allow me to launch my career in L.A. And secretly, slowly, starting to lose weight.

It's important to remember not to overlook what you love, even if you're just messing around with it. In his book, *Outliers*, Malcolm Gladwell talked about the theory that, if you invest 10,000 hours in anything, you can become an expert at it.

That's a lot of hours, but I do believe the theory applies to everybody. The trick is to make that investment of time in something that doesn't feel like hard work. You're going to have a lot more fun—and be a lot more willing to keep at it—if you actually enjoy hours 1, 2, 3, 4, and beyond on your way to becoming an expert. That's why it's so important to figure out what makes you feel really good and energized, and do more of it in your life. That's what dancing was for me: something that made me feel so good as I was doing it that I wanted to keep doing it. I had a lot of weight to lose, a lot of personal stuff to get past, and a lot of dancing to do. So, I got *busy* putting in practice time, because every hour of it made me feel better and better.

During my freshman year in college, the RAs in my dorm were getting together to do the MTV *Grind* workout, with Eric Nies and the cast of *The Real World*. It was super-big in the early 1990s. I can still feel the excitement I had when Eric ran onto the stage without a shirt, like he just happened to forget to wear one that day.

Hey, what's up everybody?

Hey, Eric! What up yourself?

He would lead his dancers in studio—and me, in my dorm—through some warm-ups and breathing exercises, sweeping his arms up over his head on an inhale, and dropping them on the exhale. Then, we'd grind out our dance moves for 20 to 30 minutes. I got sweaty and I got sore, and I loved every second of it.

By sophomore year, I was something of a gym rat, and it only made sense for me to look in on the Dancercise classes that were happening down the hall from the weight room. I was ready to step it up.

That's how I met Mandee Kern, the dope group-exercise teacher at the Rowan Rec Center. Maybe you've heard the saying: When the student is ready, the teacher appears. Well, Mandee was one of the most important people in my life, because she opened me up to all the things that dancing and exercise and being a class leader could do for me, and for others.

Mandee was a key uplifter for me.

She had jet black hair and lots of piercings and tattoos, so she was going *way* beyond Jane Fonda and her leggings. And her badass attitude was packing women into her step-and-tone class. So, I went, too. I didn't care if I was the only guy in there, I wanted to be where she was.

(Years later, she helped out on one of my *INSANITY* DVDs. When you find somebody like her, she's a good-luck charm you keep real close.)

Mandee's class used an 8-inch step to boost aerobic fitness, and hand weights to encourage muscle toning. I walked into my first class and saw all the ladies in their leotards and leg warmers, holding 2-pound dumbbells, and I thought, "Why y'all using those little-bitty weights?"

Being a guy with a big ego, I grabbed some 10-pound dumbbells and said "Okay, we ready."

Dumbbell, exactly.

Ten minutes in, I was gasping to myself: "That's what you get for being cocky, thinking you could do this!"

Mandee saw that my arms were about to fall off, so she walked over, and quietly handed me smaller weights. We instantly became friends. It was a skill of hers I admired and copied when I had the chance: Offering help without a side order of humiliation.

It might surprise you to know that the creator of *INSANITY* and *CIZE*® was a mess in his early Dancercise classes. But of course I was. I had a lot to learn. I love that about me back then. Because here's the good thing I did: I went ahead and learned, rather than running from the room.

Those of you who remember your first time through my *CIZE* workouts will know what I'm talking about. She'd go left, I'd go right and slam into a wall or the person next to me.

But, no matter how bad I was or how many mistakes I made or how frustrated I sometimes felt, I had fun. And, I kept at it. My mistakes were proof of my progress, because they showed me that I was in my discomfort zone. I was soaking up the rhythm, pouring out the sweat, and melting off my freshman 50 with so much more enjoyment than I ever had putting them on.

> **TRUTHBOMB:** Being perfect isn't the point; being *present* is.

The Domino's guy never delivered like Mandee. I just wanted more of what she was offering—the chance to move and improve, so I hardly noticed that it was a killer workout.

Every new situation is a new opportunity, and every new person you meet might change the course of your life. Look at people that way, and see how much energy you invest in new activities and chance encounters. They might be just what, or who, you need.

I THREW MYSELF INTO MY COLLEGE courses in health promotion and sports science, and I began to see my path clearly. I was Pop-Pop with his bullhorn, but instead of a street corner, I would work in an exercise studio. My gospel was exercise science, and my heavenly choir would blast out of a tape deck.

As a requirement for my major, I had to promote and teach an exercise class. So I went to the rec center and spoke with Tina Pinocci, the boss there. She asked, very reasonably: "Do you have any experience teaching?"

"No, but I can dance," I told her.

I guess I hadn't quite thought through this job interview.

"What do you want to teach?" she asked. I was afraid of tripping people's gaydar, so I told her, "I ain't teaching no high-low, no step class. I want to teach hip-hop aerobics."

I was 7 years away from when *Hip Hop Abs*® would plant my flag in the fitness industry, but even then, I knew if you could move to music *and* help people *and* lay down a six pack, why would you do it any other way?

Tina agreed.

The rec center promoted my class in the school newspaper

and on bulletin boards around the campus. And I spread the word with my big mouth.

Welcome to your discomfort zone, Shaun T!

I told everybody I knew to come.

But would they?

When I showed up at the rec center on debut day, 90 people were lined up to register.

Tina Pinocci had a big smile on her face. She'd never had *this* problem before.

"Only 60 people can fit into the room," she told me, "so you'll have to do *two classes back-to-back.*"

I had never even taught *one* class. So, why not teach 2? Or 20! This from a guy who had been afraid to walk into the weight room a few months earlier.

By all rights, I should have been scared. Instead, I was just excited. And, I was determined to prove Tina right for putting me on the schedule. I kept thinking of the Fugees song about how anything can happen when you roll into the carnival. I was going to find out if I was the guy who ran the Ferris wheel or the one who couldn't afford a ticket to ride.

I hadn't practiced at all. No curriculum, no exercise list. But the *Grind* workout was in my body and in my heart, so that part was easy.

I had my routine. Thanks, Eric Nies!

And what revolutionary music did I slap on the sound system?

"Space Jam," over and over, again and again.

Okay, my first class wasn't a Shaun T original, but once you get inside the room, it's not all about the moves. It's about what people need to motivate them that day. Since that first class, I've been able to feel the room and provide a spark, and we caught fire together right from the start.

I knew from the moment I stepped in front of the classroom that I had found my passion and my calling. Even though it was a lot of work, I could tell instinctively that there were a lot of skills required for an instructor. You have to know your music in 32-count phrases, because that's typically how the exercises will fit in well. But, you have to have a sense for that without counting 1 . . . 2 . . . 3 . . . 4 . . . 5 . . . 6 . . . 7 . . . 8 . . . out loud, or moving your lips. There's so much else going on in the group exercise room that you need to find a way to internalize the tempo of the music.

You also have to pick music that is going to complement what's happening inside the classroom and that will help everybody keep up their pace. Today, I love Baltimore Club mix to work out to, and Rihanna. My DJs can take any of her songs and create a dance mix, so it can back a workout, too. It comes down to whether the music has the right beat to drive your exercises. If it does, Shaun's going to move with it. Even if it's "Space Jam" on repeat. The music has to be clear enough and motivating enough that even the klutziest nondancer will be able to find the rhythm.

In the early days, my workout playlists were nonexistent, but I had a sense for the rhythms that would motivate movement. I knew how "Space Jam" made me feel inside, and guess what? I saw it in my students as well. The beat is a mental bond for everybody in the room, linking us together in sweat and the search for salvation. Armies march to the beat of a drum, and so do my soldiers in self-improvement!

Most important, when you're leading a class, you always have to be thinking ahead to the next steps. This is important in group exercise: prepping people to start the next step, while they're completing the current one. And being able to coach people to sync up with you, as the instructor. You have to see who's getting it, and who isn't, and kick the experts into high gear while you're coaching the newcomers *without* making them feel like idiots.

And, on top of it all, you have to reach into the soul of every person in your class and find the words to motivate them to dig deep into their reserves to find more energy, to reach for a new level, maybe even a new life. When an instructor is too focused on getting the moves right, or is only teaching to the people who already know what they're doing, a group class can quickly start feeling negative and exclusive. Every person—whether they're a professional or whether it's their first time in any group class ever—should feel like they're accomplishing something as a group, no matter how in sync they are with each other's footwork. When everybody's in it together, the energy just explodes, and everybody walks out feeling amazing. It could be chaos, or it could be the Rockettes, and it's all on the instructor to pull it off. I knew it was my job to make sure that we all got through it together.

Even in that first class, it all came as naturally to me as breathing.

I want to tell you: *I ate that class.*

People were shocked: "How long have you been teaching?"

Heck, I was a little surprised myself. I expected good things, but I admitted: "I never taught before."

A chorus answered back in disbelief: "Yes, you *have*!"

"No, that was my first time."

I did it all again immediately, because 30 more people had been waiting an hour. But I had them on that . . . I'd been waiting my whole life.

I had found my way to the front of the classroom, and I've stayed there ever since.

Soon, I got certified in kickboxing, spinning, and basic group exercise. But, the most fun I had was working with Mandee. She would train me how to teach aerobics, and I would teach her how to dance hip hop. It was one of those you-got-chocolate-in-my-peanut-butter moments, and we developed all kinds of new classes that incorporated dance in fitness, and vice-versa.

We would stay in the gym until it closed at 11:00 p.m. or

midnight, choreographing performances and dragging the rec center secretary, Joyce Pierce, out to be our audience. She was about 70 years old at that time, but she was the best audience I ever had.

You know what I was saying about making sure you have the right people around you? Recruit a Joyce Pierce for your team. Positivity is the sunlight in your garden. You won't grow without it.

Pretty soon, people from the dance department at Rowan caught on to what Mandee and I were up to, and they started attending classes as well. These people had been trained classically, or in jazz or modern disciplines, and I was just this guy from Deptford who really loved hip hop. But, I had an energy and passion that had been beaten out of dancers by teachers who were dreaming of Swan Lake, not Grandmaster Flash.

As the rec center and the dance department joined forces, Mandee and I choreographed a huge show that took the best from both disciplines. It was a hit in the community, and suddenly, we were getting invitations from local dance troupes to choreograph for them. Now I was teaching 19 exercise/dance classes every week, so my freshman 50 melted like a dropped water ice on a Jersey boardwalk.

I was also working toward my health and exercise science major, and I threw a minor in dance onto the pile. That added another year to my undergraduate career. I was on the 5-year or 10,000 hours plan, whichever came first, and making up for lost time in both dance and exercise science.

I'm still applying the lessons I learned early on in my time as an instructor. It's a great place to study how human beings build themselves up and tear themselves down. When they quit, and when they push through. Exercise is only one form of personal struggle, of course, but I've noticed that the rules that govern the gym apply pretty well across the board in life.

One of my key challenges as an instructor is determining

what 100-percent effort looks like. It's one thing for me, another for my husband, Scott, another for the lady in the back of the hall at a *Shaun T Live* event. And it changes, depending on where any of us is on our journey through life.

In fact, the person who finds the courage just to start exercising after a long lay-off—making a tentative step out the door for a walk around the block—is doing something just as heroic as the person who busts the tape at the Chicago Marathon. My mission as a trainer/motivator is to see those wonderful individual needs and accomplishments, and celebrate them, and help people feel good about them—wherever they are on the fitness spectrum.

My deepest hope for you is that you can congratulate yourself on *where you are today*, even if it's not where you ultimately want to be. If you're in the process of transformation, every step along the way is necessary to reach the final goal. So, focus on the step you're taking, invest it with all you have, and feel great about that.

What's *in* your 100 percent will change, but *the will* to push for 100 percent remains constant. That's the only victory I want to celebrate, and I hope we can celebrate it together.

MY WORLD WAS STILL PRETTY SMALL at this point, so when I went looking for a job after graduation, I set my sights on beautiful New Jersey. You can't get more Jersey than being the health-and-fitness specialist at a nuclear power plant. But, you know, people who split atoms for a living don't want to be splitting their pants as well. I was there for them, because I probably still had a few 40-inch-waist pants in my closet, too.

I can remember driving to the PSE&G plant in Salem, N.J., like it was yesterday. (I was evacuated from there after the airplanes hit the World Trade Center towers, so it's seared in my brain.) I was training engineers who spent their days staring at computer monitors and filing into the gym to do the same workouts day after day. They were in their comfort zones, alright, and suffering from it. So, my mission was to make them uncomfortable and to shake their bodies into a healthier lifestyle.

Shake their booties, too.

I didn't let up, not one tiny bit. I told them, "I don't know what y'all been doin', but I'm here now, and you're going to *move*." Bosses, employees, maintenance workers were all in the mix together, shaking stuff that hadn't been shaken for years.

I knew where they were coming from—the same place I did freshman year. So, I made sure that their lunch break really was a break—from what they had been doing that morning, and from what they'd been doing with their lives.

Eventually, I moved on to a job where progress was a corporate priority: in employee wellness at Wyeth, one of the world's largest pharmaceutical companies. I was teaching classes at a local dance studio on the side, and dancing my heart out every spare minute when I wasn't doing all that other stuff.

Sometimes, it seemed that I was either leading a class, dancing, or sleeping. I was 22 years old, give or take 10,000 hours.

Does it all seem too much to you? Like, you couldn't possibly fit anything else into your crammed life?

Well, I haven't reviewed your to-do list, so I couldn't say. But let me try something out on you. A lot of people build all kinds of busyness into their lives as a way of crowding out difficult questions.

If you're running from 6:00 a.m. until 11:00 p.m., maybe you won't have time to ask yourself whether you're running in the right direction for the right reasons.

A lot of people complain that they couldn't squeeze in the 25 minutes it takes to sweat through *FOCUS T25*. And that may be the case. But I have to ask: If the average American is watching 5 hours of television a day plus scrolling through social media, who's logging all that tube time, to push the numbers up?

What's binge-watching, without binge-ers?

Here's my suggestion: Take 3 days, and log every minute of your time. How long do you spend at work, how long commuting, how long cooking dinner, how long scrolling Facebook or Twitter, how long parked in front of the television? Then, total the time in the various categories.

My guess is that, somewhere, a giant time suck will jump out at you. And, when you cut it back, you'll open windows of time to pursue my favorite activity.

What's that?

Living in your discomfort zone, of course.

T IS FOR TRANSFORMATION

SUPERPOWER #1: UNCOMFORTABILITY

Teaching my first exercise class put me in an uncomfortable position: I'd never done that before. Perfect place to kick off a growth spurt, in fact. To develop new abilities, you need to move out beyond your comfort zone and accept that you don't have all the answers. Sometimes, you don't even know the questions! But people who are *comfortable with discomfort* perform well during life's shake-ups. They take risks and initiate change. Okay, they can be somewhat reckless. But you can be adventurous without actually diving straight off the cliff into the ocean, you know?

SELF-TEST:
HOW UNCOMFORTABLE ARE YOU?

[1 = That's me! 6 = That's totally not me!]

1. If I hear that my friend is talking behind my back, I'll still accept her invite to the movies.

1	2	3	4	5	6

2. When my boss is on the warpath, I lay low.

1	2	3	4	5	6

3. I go to the same five restaurants, and order the same five meals.

1	2	3	4	5	6

4. I haven't changed my hairdo since 2002.

1	2	3	4	5	6

5. I listen to the oldies station 24/7.

1	2	3	4	5	6

SCORE BOX

Mostly 1s and 2s: Indiana Jones, you're not.

Mostly 3s and 4s: You're more mild-ass than wild-ass.

Mostly 5s and 6s: Welcome to the jungle! (Make sure you don't get eaten out there, okay?)

SHAUN T'S
DiSCOMFORT DEVELOPMENT PLAN

EXERCISE #1

Put yourself in an uncomfortable position. It could be holding a plank for 5 minutes, or joining a sports league with players who are literally out of your league, or learning the benefits of high-intensity interval training, or committing to the 5-minute workouts I post on Facebook. If your fitness plan doesn't make you a little uncomfortable, it's probably not giving you the benefits you want. So, do this for me, as a way of flexing your new uncomfortable superpower: Push yourself to new level that makes you gasp, makes you sore, makes you wonder why Shaun T has it in for you. And then, push through to succeed at it. That breakthrough is something you can then repeat throughout your life, wherever a little dose of discomfort can serve you best.

Ask yourself: What's the worst that could happen? Trying a new food, starting a new workout plan, inviting somebody new out to lunch, taking a flyer on a job interview, or booking an Airbnb in an exotic locale might put you at risk of a bad meal, a bad night's sleep, or some sore muscles, but it could also introduce you to your new favorite thing. Discomfort is risk. Discovery is the reward for that risk.

EXERCISE #2

Find more adventurous friends. Look around at your inner circle. Are they pushing their envelopes, or sealing, licking, and stamping them firmly in place? Push outside your boundaries. Attend guest lectures by world travelers, encounter entrepreneurs at meet-up events, read books by revolutionaries. These are people who are comfortable with discomfort, and they can show you the way. You don't have to climb Everest. Just meet people who see walls and immediately want to climb over them. You never know who might boost you over to the other side.

EXERCISE #3

Boldly go. As bad as it was for me at home as a kid, I lived with the situation for nearly a decade. Even a deep, dark rut sometimes looks safer than an unknown future. But, you have to take steps into that future, especially if it's uncomfortable for you to think about it. Remember how El Chapo plotted his prison escape for months ahead of time? Well, I don't want to compare you to a South American drug kingpin, but he was onto something. If the thought of a new life makes you uncomfortable, invest time in planning. Acquire new skills for the new life. Meet the new people you'll be with when you get there. As you add details of the place you're headed, it will seem inevitable, not scary. Who's going to help *you* tunnel to freedom?

EXERCISE #4

Expose yourself to new ideas. If you're getting all the same inputs all the time—watching the same shows, reading the same books, listening to the same music, downloading the same podcasts—you'll remain stuck with all the same old ideas. You need someone to challenge your viewpoints, make you squirm. If you admire an innovator/trouble-maker at work, ask her what she's reading. If your teenager has crazy music tastes, ask him what's good. If you admire (or even loathe) a political figure, read her biography. If your girlfriend is always pushing the line on what she wears, go shopping with her.

TRUTHBOMB: If you want to change your outputs, change the inputs.

EXERCISE #5

Find a new path. I mean that literally. If you've belonged to one gym for the last 3 years, book a new membership. Go to a different coffee shop. Drive away for the weekend. Open up your own Airbnb. Remember, your comfort zone can be a death trap, if you let it be. If you literally put yourself in new (uncomfortable) places, you'll meet new (maybe important) people. I drove all the way from New Jersey to Los Angeles and found the key people out there who would show me what was possible in my new life, and also hot-wire those possibilities. Discomfort means that you're on the way! What's your Jersey? Where's your L.A.? Put your butt in the driver's seat, recruit a co-pilot with the right attitude to make sure you don't turn back, and *go*. There's no telling where you might end up!

Are You Headed Off a Cliff?

Are you strong enough to jump that gap between where you are and where you want to be? Or, will you wind up on the rocks below? The comfortable uncomfortable person practices small hops all along the way to her transformation triple-jump. Don't force change in an instant. Make it happen a little every day.

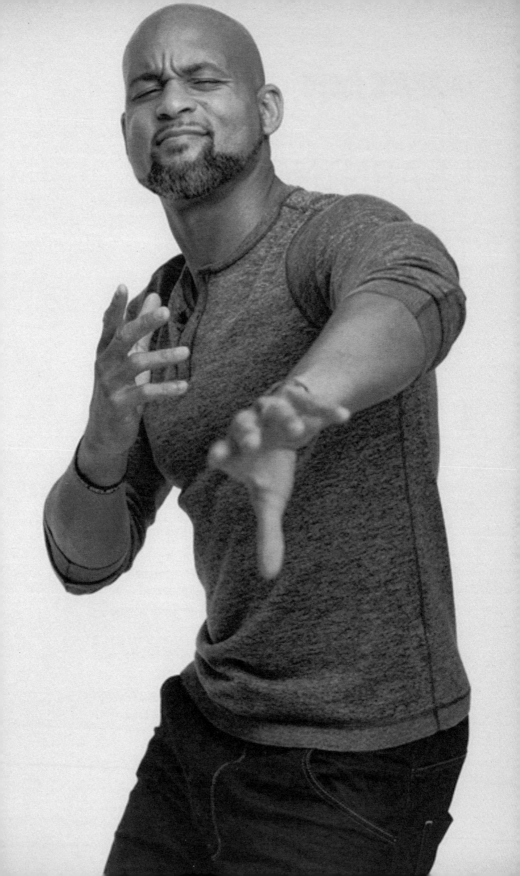

CHAPTER EIGHT

LEARNING TO LIVE IN THE EIGHTS

It's pretty common among people who have been heavy— that is, *me*—to look in the mirror and see who they used to be at their most extreme, not who they are now.

But weight isn't the only thing that causes that gap between the image you're showing the world and what you see when you look in the mirror.

Tell me if any of these gap sensations sound familiar:

You get a few promotions at work and you wear the expensive clothes that tell the world: I belong in this office. (But secretly, you doubt that you really do.)

You buy the car that says: I'm going places, and this is the ride that's going to take me there. (But only you know that you maxed out on car payments, and it's getting tricky in your checking account.)

You pull on the Lululemon workout gear that's a second skin, and show off every curve you've worked so hard to sculpt. (But underneath those clothes, you still see flaws in the yoga studio mirror, and worry that others are seeing them too.)

Upside, meet downside.

So, what's going on for you inside that the rest of the world can't see? More important, are your exteriors compensating for interiors you're not happy with? That shiny surface stuff might be sending off flashes of light to distract you from your dark places.

And I'm all about shining light into those dark places.

TRUTHBOMB: To get a healthy body, you have to start with a healthy life.

When I was in my early twenties, I had the healthy body, but I was struggling to match it against the unhealthy feelings that were still roiling inside.

I think that's why my mental image (still lugging a burden of weight around) didn't match up with the one I was showing to the world (fit dancer/teacher/badass).

That's what 21-year-old Shaun was struggling with: Where had I been, and where I was going? What kind of soiled underwear was still hiding in the closet? What kind of emotional Samsonite was I dragging around behind me? How did I view myself now?

I had tidied up the outside, yes, but on the inside, I was driven by all the stuff that I was still afraid of. I was moving alright, but I wasn't clearing hurdles, exactly. I was running away from them.

A lot of us fail to deal with the mistakes, regrets, and burdens of the past, to the extent that we live with that stuff long after we need to.

How many times do you find yourself reliving a difficult moment, and cursing yourself for what you didn't say or do to get out of it?

How many times do you react to an old wound by poking and prodding it until it bleeds again?

How many times do you keep alive an old, less-capable vision of yourself, and prop it up as an example of who you are now, instead of who you were way back when?

In dance, we have an expression called living in the eights—the eight-count that forms the backbone of most contemporary music. If you're in the eights, you're locked in with the beat and up to the moment with your reactions.

The opposite is no fun at all: Living out of sync. Living behind the beat. Missing your moment.

I know why I did that. There was so much I couldn't yet face, hadn't processed, hadn't released into the past. You can't live in the eights until you fully inhabit the present moment.

So, stop counting backward, and move your life forward.

LET ME TELL YOU ABOUT A dream I had recently, about a special lady I knew in New York. She had green skin and weighed 450,000 pounds.

That's right: Shaun T dreams about the Statue of Liberty sometimes.

Freedom has always been a big deal for me. You could say that the biggest move of my life came when I busted out of my home in search of freedom from sexual abuse. So, when Lady Liberty appears in my dreams, I suspect I'm using that to work through feelings about personal freedom.

In my dream, I was falling from the Statue of Liberty. I was like: "Oh my God. Am I going to be able to land?"

But my dream answer was the only safe one: "I'm landing this sh*t!"

They say if you hit the ground in one of those falling dreams, you actually die. But how would "they" know? Anyway, in my dream, I spread my toes, bent my knees, and came down softly. It was a perfect 10 landing.

Then, I woke up with a start, and thought: *Don't tell me I can't land!*

How are your landing skills here in the real world?

Learning to fall well is a skill all of us need to practice, especially if the Statue of Liberty herself is looking on in the background. We're only really free if we give ourselves permission to fail and to fall. We need to practice that soft landing so that we're not afraid of it, and so we can spring back up again.

I know I can do it, because I've had plenty of experience with it, both awake and asleep. In fact, that was what age 21 was like for me. I was figuring out how I could end a long, scary fall with a soft touch-down, while reserving energy for another, higher leap.

I'm not saying it was a comfortable time. Not by a long stretch. But, you know how I feel about that. I repeat: Progress begins at the end of your comfort zone.

A big part of the problem was that I was still trying to fool everybody about my sexuality. So, I must have left a lot of my girl friends (two words) wondering why they weren't my *girlfriends* (one word).

At the time, gay people were still considered oddballs, at best, and social deviants, at worst. Mariah Carey's song "Outside" was my anthem back then, and my burden. I woke up every morning to her lyrics—a comfort and support for every outsider—and felt she was singing directly to me.

It wasn't until my 4th year of college that I felt free enough to get into a legit relationship. I'd had a few hook-ups with other closeted gay men, who, like me, were covering it up pretty well. And, even when I started looking for a real boyfriend, it wasn't like I was attending single-sex mixers or parties.

Rowan probably had an LGBT coalition, but I wasn't joining it. Not ready for that. And I couldn't hook up with men who were already out of the closet, because there was always the fear that they would out me. So, on the one hand, it was a relief to feel that I could have a boyfriend and share a living space, but it was a worry that somebody might discover that we were more than just roommates. It probably seems weird to think back on those times, when people were living secret lives and fearing discovery. It was so recent, and so long ago, that I lived a lie and defended that lie in the eyes of the world.

This was no way to live, but I learned so much from it. It's like that moment in a workout where annoying Shaun T reminds you: "Don't run from the work. *Feel* the work."

My work at that time was experiencing the pain of life in the closet, so I would have motivation to bust out.

Still, I'm not sure when I would have come clean if not for Pop-Pop's intuition . . . and big mouth.

One afternoon late in my college career, when I had been living with my boyfriend for a year or so, I asked him to pick up something I'd left at my grandparents' house.

Pop-Pop was waiting for him.

"I want to talk to you about your relationship with Shaun," he began.

Uh-oh.

Mom-Mom to the rescue!

"Charles!" she shouted, "He doesn't have time for that right now. He has to go pick up his *girlfriend*."

Where she pulled that girlfriend out of, we'll never know. But my boyfriend took the opportunity to run for the door.

When he told me this story, I panicked first, and felt annoyed second. I thought: "*What* relationship? That's a big secret y'all don't know anything about!"

Or, so I imagined.

But, I knew the clock was ticking on my "secret" being all over my world. I needed to talk to Mom, pronto . . . and Ennis!

The next day, I met my mom at my grandparents' house.

The coast was clear—Mom-Mom and Pop-Pop were down-stairs—so, I told her, "We have to talk."

My heart was pounding. If this conversation went badly, it might be the last one I ever had with her. Or, it could be the start of a new level of honesty in our lives. In my life!

But which?

She sat down, looked me in the eye, and simply listened. It was one of her greatest skills, and gifts to me. Close mouth, open ears. It really works.

First up: I told her the story of how the man she invited into her house abused me for 4 years.

Once I'd spilled that, it was kind of an afterthought to say, "Oh, and by the way, I'm gay."

What a day in the life for a parent, right?

"Well, you are what you are," she said. It was kind of a shoulder shrug for her.

Bless her for that. As for the other part of our conversation, her only consolation was that that man was long gone from her life and that I had survived.

On to Ennis. I swore my mother to secrecy—"Do not tell Ennis!"—and arranged to meet my brother after work the next day.

The first minute I saw him, he said: "Mom already told me. You're gay. Whatever. Let's get something to eat."

And nothing I could ever say would shock him about the stepmonster. He'd assumed the worst about that guy from the beginning and barely spoke 12 words to him his entire life. That shows you how smart Ennis was.

In the end, coming out wasn't such a big revelation after all. And why should it be? Have you ever heard of anybody coming out as heterosexual? It's just assumed, we are who we are. I rest my case.

Coming out as a gay man, I knew that certain people were going to immediately dislike me. So, was I going to hide myself forever because certain people might disapprove?

That's when I made a vow: I ain't hiding nothing else. I did that as a kid, I damn sure ain't doing that as an adult. No, if you don't accept me, fine. The people who love me accept me.

TRUTHBOMB: Most important: I accept me. You can't do better than that.

TRUTHBOMB: You're imprisoned by what you hide, because that means *you* haven't accepted it. Honesty frees you to be *you*.

Just ask Lady Liberty.

WHILE WE'RE TALKING ABOUT BREAKING FREE, let me tell you about the time Janet Jackson tied me to her bondage table.

My college boyfriend knew I was a huge Janet fan—I had the official JJ T-shirt!—so for my birthday, he bought us tickets to her concert in Philly. But, when we showed up at the venue, primed for an amazing time, the usher told us that there was something wrong with the tickets, and we were sent over to the ticket office. The ticket guy got one look at broken-hearted Shaun and made a decision that this guy deserved to be closer to the stage.

He stood up and gestured, "Follow me."

We popped out of this little office, and walked the aisle toward the stage, passing rows and rows of people who had paid hundreds to be there. He inserted us into the second row, so we'd be breathing the same air as Janet.

I couldn't believe my luck. And, it was only just beginning.

Janet's concerts back then featured one song—"Would You Mind"—with some memorable audience participation. We kind of got to know the people around us in row two, and they could feel my Jackson love. So, they all pledged to offer me up when Janet was choosing her victim that night.

Except when Janet said, "It's kind of lonely up here on the stage"—her teasing intro to "Would You Mind"—they all went berserk, trying to attract her attention. I stood quietly, locked eyes with her, and broadcast my message: "Girl, it's just you and me."

Janet milked her decision for a good minute, stalking the stage in her black leather and stilettos. But, she finally returned my gaze and pointed: "I want him." Her bodyguards grabbed me under the armpits and lifted me into Heaven. Janet took my hand and walked me over to a bondage table at the center of the stage.

Fifty shades of Shaun, y'all!

She cinched the restraints around my wrists and ankles, and then she lap danced me to within an inch of heterosexuality. When the song and her writhing seduction ended—the fastest, and longest, 4 minutes of my life—Janet kissed me on the cheek and said "thank you." Then Shaun and his bondage chair dropped beneath the stage, riding some kind of elevator platform. The crowd roared as I disappeared.

Down in the dungeon, a technician freed me. Then, he handed me a Polaroid of Shaun, center stage, looking incredibly grateful that he'd received the wrong tickets for the most exciting night of his life.

It took us forever to clear the stadium that night; everybody wanted to take a picture of the guy Janet Jackson strapped to a table. My cell phone exploded with congratulations.

Janet Jackson did *what* to you?

WHICH BRINGS ME BACK TO MY boyfriend. You'd think he would have been glad for me. He'd arranged this amazing date, and look at all that had come from it. Instead, in his eyes, the evening was just another example of Shaun getting all the attention. He wasn't glad for me; he resented it.

After Janet released me from my shackles, I released myself as well. Once I came out to my mom and Ennis, I knew I needed to be out of that relationship as well.

Right around this time, I danced in a showcase at the Garden State Dance Festival. This wasn't Broadway. It wasn't even a West Side strip club on Manhattan. No dressing rooms, no privacy, no time for modesty. Dancers were flinging clothes and costumes off right under each other's noses. So, there I was nearly naked in a room with 20 women, and the other dancers were like "Check out Shaun T. He got *abs*!"

In 3 years, I'd gone from candy-coated to eye candy. It was a whole new kind of liberation: The freedom to feel proud about my body and myself.

Did you hear that, Lady Liberty?

The showcase was one of the best nights of my life.

Suzy Zucker was the lead choreographer of the festival. She insisted on strict professionalism and high standards, two superpowers I would pack away for my trip to L.A. in a couple of years. She admired my work ethic, took me under her wing, and let me assist her for the show. I wasn't about to blow that opportunity.

I choreographed a dozen dancers to "The End," by Linkin Park, and the audience's response blew me away. The more they cheered, the higher I jumped and the more energy I gave back. It was a defining moment for me. I'd spent years losing weight, teaching dozens of classes, and rising up as a dancer, and now I was able to put it on stage for everybody to see.

It was the best. The best. The *best*.

But not everybody enjoyed the show.

In fact, it was the last thing my soon-to-be ex-boyfriend wanted to hear about when I got home after the show. A confident Shaun wasn't going to put up with his stuff, and he knew it.

I remember exactly what he said to me that night. "You can be as happy as you want, but you're never going to be a professional dancer."

To this day, if you really want to motivate me, just tell me what I can't do.

Step one toward my next life was to clear the hurdles from my current one. My boyfriend was one of them.

I planned my exit. One day while the boyfriend was away I called Ennis and said, "Help me bounce from this place." We packed up all my clothes in trash bags and I made my getaway. My path forward was clear at last.

TRADITIONAL MARRIAGE VOWS ARE FILLED WITH "until death do us part" and "for better or worse," but they don't say anything about how you are going to change over the course of your lifetimes. Your partner is going to change, too.

You need to be clear about changes as they're happening, and encourage your partner to do the same. You have to accept where they want to go, what they want to do, and who they want to be. The same goes for you. With that mutual support, your relationship can improve through the changes.

But, if someone isn't accepting your path—husband, wife, lover, friend, boss, parent—they aren't accepting you. It's similar to what I was going through back in my closeted days.

TRUTHBOMB: We're all in the closet about something.

The energy we spend being something other than who we are is a total waste. We could be out in the world living our truths, rather than hiding among our lies.

What are you in the closet about, and why?

Are you afraid the haters will target you? Afraid that the people close to you won't accept who you really are, rather than who you're pretending to be for their benefit?

Don't let them grab that power.

If you do, you'll be living your life for people who love a make-believe you. Come clean about the real you to the people in your circle who really matter, because they'll support you for who you really are.

Your happiness will become their happiness.

Your freedom will make them more free.

Anybody who doesn't feel that way?

Leave them behind you as you move forward.

SELF-TEST:
HOW STRONG IS YOUR CIRCLE OF FIVE?

In his book *The Slight Edge*, Jeff Olson presents his theory that each of us is the average of the five people who are closest to us. That is, our personal identities are kind of a combo pack of the strengths and weaknesses of our closest circle of friends, relations, and even enemies. That can be a great thing, unless—as various toxic people in my life have proved—it's awful.

Who's dragging you under?

Who's pulling you up?

And do you have enough uppers, and can you lessen the impact of the downers?

The more I thought about the Big Five people, the more I began to wonder if there was an even more useful way to look at them. Not just identify them, but ask yourself how negative or positive an influence are they on your life, and what can you do to turn the negatives into positives?

Or, shut the negatives down altogether?

You inherit the energy around you, whether you like it or not.

Use this exercise to turn your minuses to pluses.

THE "BIG FIVE" TEST

Write down the five people who affect your life the most right now. It could be your mom, your boss, or your boyfriend, girlfriend, husband, or wife. This isn't a history exercise. Draw the circle tight and current.

1. _____

2. _____

3. _____

4. _____

5. _____

Negative/positive ratings

On a scale of 1 to 10, how positive an influence are they in your life? (Ten means that they are to positivity what the sun is to a cornfield, and 1 means that they're a black hole of negativity—chilly, dark, an emotion-sucker. A 5 means sometimes good, sometimes bad.)

1. _____

2. _____

3. _____

4. _____

5. _____

Can you help them improve?

Again, on a scale of 1 to 10, write down how much of an effect you can have on these people. Are they open to conversation? If they are a negative influence, have you tried to change the dynamic? If they're actively asking for more from you, like your kids would, that's a 10. And, maybe your employee is a 5, if she's causing problems, but looking for feedback, too.

1. _____

2. _____

3. _____

4. _____

5. _____

Can they help you improve?

Now, rank them 1 to 10 on how positive an influence they can be in your life. If your boss is trouble, but really knows her stuff and is willing to teach, maybe she rates an 8. If your miserable sister-in-law can only demonstrate how to talk mean and eat cheese puffs, she's a 1 or 2.

1. _____

2. _____

3. _____

4. _____

5. _____

Communication score

How well do you communicate with these five people? Ten is: We can talk about anything. One is: Might as well talk to the wall. Maybe they refuse to listen, or maybe you really struggle to figure out how to talk to them about what's most important to you.

1. _____

2. _____

3. _____

4. _____

5. _____

The Math

Add up your numbers, and divide by two.

Your "Big Five" Number

Where'd you come out? Read it like a school teacher would.

60 or less	F
61–70	D
71–80	C
81–90	B
91–100	A (and you can teach this course yourself.)

I never do much better than around 85 on this test, even though Scott is pulling my number way up. But then, there are all those Felicias out there—the ones I need to say bye to. They're pretty much the anti-Scotts. So, I'm not exactly acing this class, either. But I'm aware and constantly communicating to elevate my score. I understand why: We so often feel stuck with the relationships we have. It's really hard to fix them, and it's equally hard to imagine ending them, so we accept the status quo, even if it includes people we wish we'd never gotten involved with. This test will let you know if your Core Five is failing you, or you are failing them, and what you can do about it.

Here are a few ways to raise your score (and improve your life).

Jack up the communication. A lot of times, when we have a difficult relationship with someone, we play dodgeball: we jump left to avoid negative comments, jump right to skip a tough talk. But then nothing changes. Sometimes, if you make the first gesture—"How are you feeling?" "How do you see this problem?" "What can I do to help you more?"—you can build your own breakthrough. If that turns a 2 into a 7, you're done playing dodgeball, and recruiting new teammates for your team. But, if they don't even realize that you were playing a game—and they think everything is fine as it is—then you know it's time to take your ball and go home.

Set the example yourself. I think about this a lot with kids. Sometimes, parents are so caught up in judging their kids, offering advice, and giving orders, that they don't think about what example they're setting. Your kid won't listen to you, huh? Are you listening to her? Your kid lies around on the couch all the time eating chips? How active are you, and who's buying those chips, anyway? Improvement works better when it's a group activity, not a Sermon on the Mount. Likewise, among us grown-ups, too often, we try to one-up our enemies with increasingly bad behavior. Maybe setting a good example could set off more positive movement. Even if it doesn't, at least one of you will be behaving properly, right? Bonus points if it's you.

Know your role. Rivalry and envy often get in the way when we're looking at somebody else's success story. So, try to step back a bit. Are you mad at her because she did you wrong or because she has something you want? Well, how did she get it? Can you use the same strategies? Can you learn her skills? And, how would your relationship change if, instead of giving her the cold shoulder, you asked for advice? Turn your rival into a mentor, and see where it gets you. And, if she won't mentor you, use her as an example, and identify someone who will. Find, then grab, a hand up.

Accept help. If you have an especially tough relationship, recruit allies. That doesn't mean building a posse of bullies to beat up your enemy. Pull aside some of the 7s, 8s, and 9s on your list, and ask them how they'd handle your situation. At the very least, you'll gain support, and, at the best, you may gain new strategies to handle the troublemaker, and to raise your own game.

Turn 2s into 6s. Are their numbers low because they have such a strong influence on you, or because you have a sore spot you invite them to punch? Maybe your dad keeps nagging you because he thinks you're capable of doing more with your career. Sure, that's annoying, but that doesn't mean you shouldn't be shoring up the weak spots on your résumé. Set aside the emotion, and look at the content of your clash. Maybe there's a to-do list in there that can move you and him up the scale.

Cut 'em loose. Are you giving too much power to the irritators? They can act however they want to, but only you determine how you'll react. Move on with your life. It really is your choice.

Make sure that your "Big Five" are the *right* five. Yes, that's a heavy suggestion. It might mean looking for a new job after you fire your boss. Maybe you need to end a relationship. Maybe you need to back off from certain "friends" and pay more attention to the ones with actual benefits. That can hurt. But, before you do any of that, use the clues in the other rankings—especially the one about communication—to face the weak spots in your Big Five. If you reach out, they may reach back. If not, better to make a painful break than suffer for a lifetime. Don't be a victim. One way to upgrade your Big Five might be to move somebody new into it, and somebody old and destructive out of it.

BONUS EXERCISE

How to Answer a Hater

While you're identifying your Core Five, you might be able to use a little quick maintenance on the worst elements around you. You know that term "resting bitch face"? We can all be that way sometimes, just waiting for other people to screw up so we can call them on it. But, let me confess straight off, I've been a hater, too, even though I own and wear the T-shirt "I'm Allergic to Haters." So, I try to stamp it out whenever I see it in myself, or others. Hater-ism—if that's a word—is the same as gossip, and it usually has a lot more to do with the person who's doing the hating than the target of their mean messages. Personally, I can't be bothered to worry about them. Why give them that power? But, I get it. Haters have a way of worming into your brain and taking up residence. How to evict them from that precious space? I've used every strategy, so I'll guide you through them.

The Shrugger. Haters gain power from your pain. If they sense that you're hurt, they're like a shark who smells blood. They're going to rip into it. But, if you treat them like the minnow they really are, you rob them of power. So, the written shrug—Hey, good luck with that—can get you out of the situation without any emotional investment.

The Hugger. Sometimes, you can shock someone into civility by reacting not to the poisonous message, but to the pain underneath it: "Wow, sounds like your problems go a lot deeper than me. Hope you find some help with them."

The Cooler. Hate is a hot emotion. It tries to light the fire, then stand in the hot glow. Be as cool as they are hot. "Wow, I didn't know you felt that way. Oh, well."

The Motivator. If you look beyond the hateful message to the motivation behind it, and make a recommendation, you might score some points with the more reasonable people. You could say, "It sounds like you have trouble dealing with people like me. But, I'm not the only one out there. If you broaden your world, you can invite a lot more people into it."

The Listener. The last thing a hater expects is to actually be taken seriously. So, when the rude comment pops up, sometimes you can shame the commenter by actually taking him/her/it seriously. "Why do you feel that way?" might not cause a hater to melt into self-reflection. Then again, it might. And, it allows you to rise high, high above abusive language into the realm of people who actually care about others.

The Tribe Builder. This is my favorite defense mechanism, because it unifies the very best people. If a friend is under attack, I give them support. Then the people who belong in my life—the ones who really listen, and share their support—jump in as well. We reinforce ties in our community and defend it. And, that's as good a reason as any to recruit friends and supporters—to find your group and create a force-field of positivity.

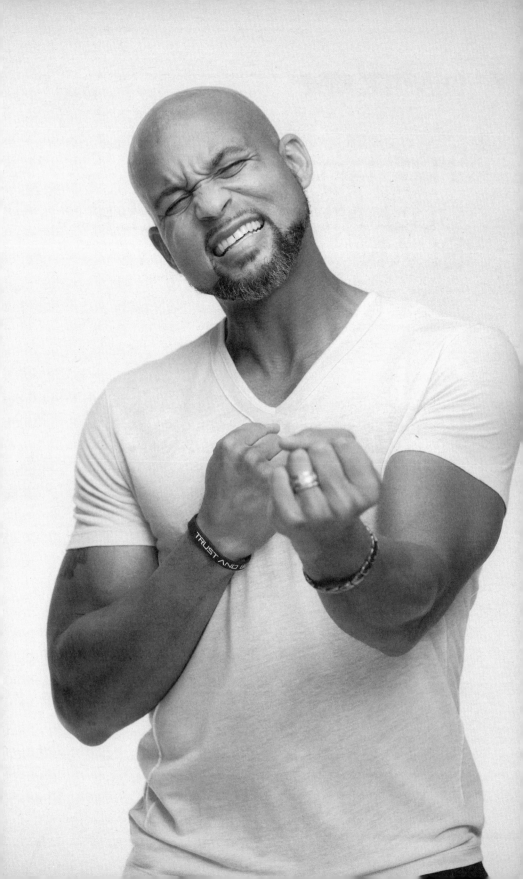

CHAPTER NINE

THE HOT-DOO-DOO-MESS CAREER PLAN

L et's listen to the soundtrack of your life for a minute.
     You don't need to cue a playlist.

It isn't music that's playing, it's all the words that you've spoken or thought in the stream of your experience.

They can be kind words you've spoken to close friends and loved ones, words you've spat out in anger against enemies, lies you told your mom when you sneaked out after midnight at age 16. (Yeah, Shaun T knows about that, too.) It can be the hopeful things you told yourself about your motives, your progress, your intentions. It could be what you told yourself as you picked up this book at the bookstore: *Maybe reading this will help me discover the best in me.* (Or, maybe it was: *I failed at that diet book I read. This one won't help me either.*)

Some people call it self-talk or your inner voice. This is where mental barriers begin; it's also where you can end them.

As you rewind your life soundtrack, you're bound to hear some sour notes. Listen carefully for the clinkers that you hear over and over again—not just the one-off misses, but the patterns of the off-notes.

You must identify these patterns and how they consistently screw up your life, and also recognize the soundtrack that was playing just before things went haywire.

Maybe it's the lies you tell yourself (and others) just to get through another day, another month, another year.

The ways you talk down your abilities by reminding yourself of every time you dropped the ball or left the field before the end of the game.

The ways you downgrade your own prospects, playing a sad soundtrack of failure that keeps you from even trying.

Those are the notes that might be holding you back from the changes you want to make in your life. So, as you commit to transformation, commit to a soundtrack that gives you credit for what you've done, that motivates you to try harder, that gives you permission to both fail *and* succeed.

This is the playlist of your life, and you control it. Ultimately, you'll dance to the music you cue up. Make sure they're *your* greatest hits. Turn it into marching music. Step out and face your problems, and don't be quiet about it!

People will try to program your music for you, of course. Maybe your officemates want you to sing in the chorus, rather than be a headliner. Maybe your parents want you to just plug into the family playlist rather than march to the beat of your own drum. Maybe they want it to be less about what you want in life, and more about what they need to get from you.

My advice is: Be the DJ. Control the playlist. Cue your future by hearing it now.

MY SOUNDTRACK WAS LOUD, BUT CONFUSED. A lot of it was danceable, but there were awkward echoes that held me back.

My act played well locally, and I didn't know if it would ever bust out of my narrow world.

My friend Herb could hear music that wasn't evident to me just yet. He suggested that I visit him in L.A., where he'd moved after college. And he said: Oh, by the way, get some headshots done. He even had a photographer for me.

Evidently, he saw something in me that my ex-boyfriend didn't—that people in L.A. might one day care who this Shaun T guy is.

I wasn't thinking that way, honestly.

My soundtrack played such golden oldies as: "Do you look good, really?" "Is that puffed up dude in the mirror really gone for good?" And the recurring hit: "Maybe your ex-boyfriend was right!"

On top of all that, my life in Jersey was pretty good: I was earning a living doing what I loved, and my journey had already carried me from a 50-pound weight-gain to a strong and good-looking core that I never could have predicted. I could have continued down that Garden State pathway for the rest of my life, familiar tunes on the CD player, and been perfectly happy. And then, none of y'all would have ever heard of Shaun T.

But, on Herb's suggestion, I went and scheduled the headshots anyway. You never know, right?

So, I drove north to meet a photographer—*You're Shaun who? From where?*—in New York City. I helped him lug his gear up five stories to the rooftop of a building in lower Manhattan. On command, I flashed and flexed for the camera, because that's what you do when you're straight outta Camden, right?

It's fairly amazeballs to think that the photos he took that day would one day end up a) on a gay dating site, posted by a guy who must have hoped to meet men with bad eyesight, and b) in the hands of Mariah Carey, who would tap on it with a well-manicured fingernail and say, "I want to dance with *him*."

More on that later.

But the way I see it, those roof-top photos are kind of like a Bible story Pop-Pop used to tell, from the book of Matthew, about the mustard seed. Sometimes, a tree grows from a speck you can barely see with the naked eye.

At the time, I was that speck, and I couldn't imagine the tree or where it would root and branch. I was okay with that. It was enough for the moment that I had cleared a path forward.

Stepmonster. Conquered.

Weight gain. Lost.

Sexual confusion. No longer!.

Closet. Cleaned out.

Disbelieving boyfriend. *Ex*-boyfriend.

I'd overcome it all by pushing through my fears, by reviewing my options, and by choosing the path of change, even when it was hard. With a track record like that, what hurdles could L.A. set up that I couldn't knock down or leap over?

My discomfort zone set my agenda, and I worked through it.

When you work through *your* discomfort zones, you're laying down superpowers that you can apply to the next challenges that pop up in your life. One success leads to another, and pretty soon, you have a winning streak going.

When you notch the victory, repeat the process. Even with some losses in there, you just might accumulate some W's that change your season around.

WHEN THE PHOTOGRAPHER SENT MY HEADSHOTS, they documented a guy I didn't really recognize. That's the magic of photo editing. He picked the images that showed me from my best angles, projecting a confidence that I didn't yet own.

The images were authentic, but they lied, because they presented a guy I hoped to be, rather than one I felt like I actually was. Still, I packed them up anyway, because why not? I flew out to L.A. on Spirit Airlines. I was the longest of long shots. But, if I wouldn't bet on me, who would? Plus, it was a round-trip ticket. Nothing to lose, except another 6 hours on a flying Greyhound bus.

I wasn't nervous or feeling overextended. I was in the right place at the right time, growing at the right pace. I was making one step at a time toward my goals—I didn't feel like I was in a race against anybody and was just enjoying each new milestone as I reached it. It was undiscovered country; every step was a success. That's what I mean when I lean into the TV screen on *FOCUS T25*® and say: "You have to do this at your own pace. Do what's right for you, and you'll be getting the same benefits as anybody who is working out here with me."

I've heard people criticize that. Saying, well, that's not really in the spirit of digging deeper—getting to the next level, and ramping it up until you reach body perfection. My response: People who try to do that will just keep ramping it up until they reach misery, and then quit. And then order three cheeseburgers just to spite me.

And, honestly, perfection is a lousy goal. If you're getting 100 percent on every test, you need to take more difficult courses. Perfection *should* be short-lived, as you find new things to improve on.

And where will you find those things?

In your discomfort zone, of course!

Heading west with pictures of that stranger from the rooftop—me, but not me!—was comfortably uncomfortable. I was excited by the possibilities for new experiences, but not expecting anything in particular. I was open to success, open to failure, open to learning from either of those outcomes. It's not a bad approach to any new venture you undertake.

Success and failure go together, because each of them is a sign of something important—*You're trying!*

I'm crazy about tennis, so let's look at it in terms of that sport. There were 6 years when Roger Federer was one of the best players in the game. But, on his way to winning 18 Grand Slams, he also lost 10. And, before he won the 2017 Australian Open, he hadn't won a Grand Slam final since Wimbledon back in 2012!

Five years of failure? I don't think so.

More like 5 years of never giving up.

My girl Serena Williams is in my opinion the best tennis player of all time, male or female. But in the early 2000s, she went through a tough time with injuries, and people began to question how bad she really wanted it.

Did she give up?

Never.

It's crazy for *anybody* to compare himself or herself to Roger or Serena. But they had downtimes along their journeys, too. It's twisted logic when we expect perfection from ourselves when even Roger and Serena have to work constantly at it.

Comparisons are trouble, in general.

Are you the tallest person in the world? Are you the shortest person in the world? Are you the prettiest person in the world? Are you the unprettiest person in the world? I have a friend who ran the New York City Marathon. Cool, right? Nine people finished the exact same second he did (4:12:51). Was he worse than the people who finished a second earlier? Better than the 11 people who finished a second later?

There's *always* going to be somebody doing better (or worse) than you are, so the comparisons have to stop with you.

The questions that you should ask yourself have nothing to do with the woman on the next treadmill over at the gym, or in your social circle, or in your imagination. If you're feeling unsure of where you are, that's okay. That's what being in your discomfort zone feels like, and as you know, that's where the real growth will happen. Ask yourself: "Am I capable of doing more? Will it make me feel better if I do?"

Come up with two yeses, and your course is clear.

Use that measuring stick as your guide, and you're bound to become really good at *something*, if you work at it hard enough.

My early confidence wasn't about bragging or having a big head. It came from the way I approached things. Early on, I identified the best way for me to think about a new skill or passion. When an interest would pop up—football, or track, or singing, or dancing, Chuck E. Cheesing, or fitness-class leading— I'd ask myself: "Is this what I really want to do?"

If the answer was "yes," I plotted a path to succeed. Only then did I set off in a new direction. I never assumed that I'd be a success. But, I knew that if I took my time to figure out the best way for me to approach a new goal from the onset, there was a good chance that I could reach it.

I wasn't the most promising candidate for Hollywood. Rowan U wasn't exactly Juilliard, and Eric Nies wasn't Baryshnikov. I was a scruffy Jersey kid, but I had a body of work not many other dancers could claim. I mean that literally. I'd been working out for a living, so I wasn't a thin ballet guy. I actually *had* a muscular body! And choreographers were looking for that when I hip-hopped onto that scene.

Of course, when I showed up, they weren't looking for it from *me*.

Another college friend was working for a rental car agency in L.A. when I arrived, so he cut me a sweet deal—free!—on a car that Enterprise didn't really want to pick you up in. So, I was mobile and free to look around for dance classes. Why not add some L.A. moves to my Jersey repertoire?

I pulled my rental beater up in front of the Millennium Dance Complex in Studio City in May 2000. I wasn't just a fish out of water, I wasn't even near the right ocean. But, something drove me through the door that day, just as it had when I entered the weight room back at Rowan, or stepped in front of my first class at the rec center. Sometimes, you just need to bust the move and see if it busts you back.

Here's where the move took me: My photo is now hanging on a wall in the lobby on Ventura Boulevard, along with other people who started their dance careers there. Thank you, Millennium, both for posting the photo and for what happened in class that day. I was a new face, with new energy, so after class, my instructor mentioned that the Clear Talent Group was holding an open audition right next door.

Maybe I wanted to drop by?

Of course! Free dance class!

Really, that's how I looked at it. Of course, I had no chance, but at least I could work up a sweat and take a glimpse down the road at where I might be if I moved to L.A. one day. The plane ticket in my pocket was like a "get out of anxiety free" card. Nothing to stress about. Going back east in a few days.

I walked into the audition space and saw the 200 other dancers who showed up. That set my heart racing. They were hip, funky, professional people, and they'd clearly been in this room before. I had no idea if I belonged in this city, let alone this audition. And that was just half the challenge, because in the front of the room I saw the high-powered agents. People with contacts. People who could secure high-profile gigs for dancers.

So, there Shaun was, a gym rat in full Jersey regalia, with my wife-beater tank and sweated-out green capri pants. Green, right, just like me. My New Balance sneakers had a hole in them.

In short, I was a hot-doo-doo mess—more a candidate to be hauled out by security than to receive professional representation. I just hoped that I could hang in there long enough to work up a sweat.

Then the audition began.

OutKast's "The Way You Move" blasted out of the speakers, which I took as a good omen. That was *my* soundtrack, and now anything was possible.

Immediately, I was *in* it!

As the music rocked on, they cut a few dancers, and we danced some more. Then they cut a few more, and we danced some more. I was focused on the music, they were focusing on clearing the dance floor. Soon, I had room to roam. It felt *good*.

It was a typical dance studio, lined with mirrors. Most of the dancers were watching themselves closely in the glass, dancing with themselves, judging their work, as they'd been trained to do. I was afraid to look up, for fear that I'd see dancers who were much better than I was. Instead, I locked in with the groove, lived in the eights, and broadcast my message: "Come for *me*! Regardless of whether you like me or not, I'm *dancing*, and you're going to know who I am before I leave here."

Before I knew it, this crowded room was narrowed down to six contenders and one Jersey guy who didn't know any better. I was one of the last dancers standing, which was the dream of 199 people who showed up that day.

And then, they dismissed us. I left behind my headshot and headed for the airport.

I still had no intention of moving to L.A. at that moment. Why would I do that?

I had a good job at home, and all my family and friends were back in Jersey. I had no worries, and no expectations.

A few days later I was standing in a laundromat in Deptford, feeding quarters into the washing machine. My cell phone lit up with an unfamiliar area code. I almost didn't pick it up. Who wants to talk to a wrong number?

It still spooks me to think about that. Answer the damn phone, T! Destiny is calling!

I barked into my phone, like "Who's *this*?"

It was my future on the line. Clear Talent Group wanted to represent me, and when could I be available for auditions?

"I'll call you back and let you know," I said, and hung up the phone. Did I even say thank you, I wonder?

Next, I called up my mom. Isn't that what you do at that moment? She didn't hesitate for a second: "If you don't go out there, you're going to regret it."

She understood my position better than I did.

I didn't have the credentials, but I was being judged by my passion, my physicality, my drive, and okay, by the deep, authentic throb of Jersey I was spewing all over the place. Sometimes, a holey New Balance can stomp the crap out of a toe shoe if you're on the right dance floor.

In fact, that OutKast song tapped into something important for me—the personal soundtrack that has been accompanying me through everything I do in life. The lyrics to that song, the beat, the way it made me feel when I was dancing in front of people who would change my life, all added up into a transformation moment.

I was ready for it.

I had earned it.

I deserved it.

And, I made it happen.

I didn't say to myself: "Shaun, these dancers are way better than you are, so just step aside and let them on through."

Instead, I was hearing this loud and clear, both from OutKast and myself: "*I like the way you move.*"

The old soundtrack was finally being recorded over. The old one. The one full of negativity.

For all of the downbeat songs on my personal soundtrack, I built a positive answer. Each accomplishment added new, successful tunes to my personal playlist.

So "The Way You Move" wasn't just a song to dance to. It was my new way of life.

I want to help you rewrite and re-record your soundtrack,

so you like the way you move as well. I want you to walk into any room playing the music of belonging, and not worrying about whether anybody has better training, better contacts, or better moves than yours.

If you have a beautiful brain and heart, the rest will take care of itself.

TRUTHBOMB: Fit doesn't have a number.

It's never about the workout itself. It's about what drives you to press play, and how you feel afterward. And, more generally, how you respond when you're faced with something really difficult. When you hear me say, "The work doesn't begin until you get tired," I could be talking about any kind of work.

The work you do when you reach out to a difficult person in your life.

The work you do when you try to master a new skill.

The work you do when you look for a job that will call on more of your capabilities.

When you get exhausted from any of that, and *then* find the will to push through, that's when great things happen for you.

I wish more people would go into the next step in their journeys—fitness or otherwise—without putting unreasonable pressure on themselves.

Not expecting success.

Not fearing failure.

Not stressing out.

Just being you, and moving forward.

That's difficult for people, especially with a fitness program.

Most people are trying to do two things: First, trying to achieve an unrealistic goal they set for themselves. Like: "I want to get back to where I was in high school." They also start comparing themselves to different people. "I want to look like that girl in the front row of my fitness class," or "I want Jennifer Lopez's booty."

And, while it is a wonder of nature, you need to leave Jennifer's booty alone! When you see it on a magazine, it has probably been airbrushed to perfection!

Forget about time-traveling back to who you were in high school. That person ain't coming back. And thank goodness for that, because you don't want that big hair anymore, anyway.

When you start a fitness journey—or any journey, really—the thing you say on the very first step should be, "I'll do the best I can at this moment, and see how that feels. I won't worry about the person next to me because they have different parents, they have a different metabolism, they have different stresses. I focus on the body I have now because I'm a new person now, with a whole lot more life under my belt. My goal is to push myself hard in this moment and enjoy what happens next."

If you can keep the focus on *your* needs, how *you* feel before, after, and during a workout or a workday, you'll be that much further down the road to the life that works for *you*.

I DIDN'T MARCH STRAIGHT INTO A career as a dancer and exercise coach in L.A. First, I had to disentangle myself from my life in New Jersey. And I was going to abandon all that based on—what?—a phone call from some dude who was going to take a percentage of paid dance gigs I hadn't landed yet? It would take a bigger leap than any I'd ever attempted on the dance floor.

I gave 2-months' notice at Wyeth, thinking I could prevent a jam at work and stockpile some paychecks at the same time. My life savings stood at about $3,000 when I went west.

Mom-Mom also helped out. She and I scraped together enough to buy the used Ford Focus that would carry me across the country. Okay, the rearview mirror was taped in place, but who wanted to look back, anyway?

People who have done my *FOCUS T25* workouts are probably rolling their eyes, thinking about me actually *driving a Focus*. I never shut up about focus during that workout, because I wanted people to give me their very best effort for the full 25 minutes. Focus is what gets you past the pain and drives you forward in life. By focusing on my dreams and my ambitions, I was able to say goodbye to friends, family, coworkers, mentors, and people who believed in me, and move to a place where I knew hardly anybody. Even if your Focus is the kind manufactured by Ford, it can take you to a whole new place. It was time for Shaun to live for Shaun and see what he could make of himself.

A narrow focus on me—my skills, my needs, my dreams— could broaden into a whole wide wonderful world, if I got the details right.

It was a Saturday afternoon when my brother, Ennis, and I hit the accelerator and pointed my car—I called her Focusina— toward the West. It was crazy. I was leaving everything I had ever known.

But I wasn't nervous. More excited than anything.

I had my launchpad ready to go. Ennis found me a room in an apartment on a roommate-finder web site. And, I had already landed a job. I'd been presenting at the ECA World Fitness Conventions almost since I started working as a teacher— no, *not* shy—and I'd humbly accepted an award as "best rising star." Don't be confused by that prize. It was an honor, not an Oscar. But through the connections I'd made at the conference I'd been able to get a job teaching at Equinox in L.A. I wouldn't be flat broke, at least.

As soon as we'd emptied my car, Ennis was off with friends, and a few days later, he flew back to Jersey. Now, it was just me and Focusina, seeing what we could make of life in Los Angeles.

Equinox paid me $50 an hour to teach a class, and pretty soon I was teaching 10 classes a week, pulling in $500, and spending only $300 a month for my room. I was living the dream, right?

Mind you, this dream included an air mattress with a hole in it.

The room I'd rented was unfurnished. I threw an exercise mat down on the floor to sleep on. After my first paycheck, I could afford the upgrade to a queen-size blow-up mattress. But there must have been a pin on the floor, or a busted seam, because my bed developed a slow leak.

I'd pump the mattress just before bedtime, and then the mattress would slowly deflate all night long. Every morning, I'd wake up on the hard floor in that room, and know it was time to teach another class.

That mattress is a great reminder of what's really important. I could have turned that hard floor into a negative piece of soundtrack.

You'll never make it in L.A., Shaun. Look at this lousy room you're living in, on this mattress that bottoms out every night. Why don't you go back to Jersey where you're comfortable, before your dreams deflate just like that lousy mattress?

Instead of that, I was asking more important questions.
Who am I?
What do I believe in?
What is my power?
Where does my power come from?
Where does my strength come from?
Where do my weaknesses come from?

While I looked for answers to those questions, I worked hard at my classes, and I met people every day who convinced me that I was on the right track.

From the beginning, my career mantra was: "If I can help even one person feel the way I did when I lost those first 4 pounds, it will be worth it."

There were hundreds of people attending my exercise classes every week, and they multiplied my passion for teaching.

There was the 40-year-old guy who came up to me after class and told me, "You've changed my life."

There was the young mom who told me, "You're helping me in a way that nobody has before."

And their teacher was sleeping on a mattress that let him down slowly every night.

CHAPTER TEN

SHAUN T, THE MUSICAL

Human beings are social animals. That's why so many of us opt to live in cities, and why the founder of Facebook is worth more than you or I would make in fifteen lifetimes. We flock together, for better or worse.

We all know the "worse" part. I want you to concentrate on maxing out the "better" part of the equation.

Back in Chapter Eight I had you review your circle of five. Some people were probably a net positive effect on your life, some negative. Think of the positive ones as your tribe. I want you to build yours into an unbeatable force. Sometimes you'll need to rely on them for support, for suggestions, for honest feedback, or maybe a couple of bucks to tide you over while you launch your can't-miss-taco-stand-and-sushi food truck. And sometimes they'll need all of that from you.

But being vulnerable, and admitting your needs, plays just as big a part as your personal strengths in attracting the right tribe.

> **TRUTHBOMB:** Admitting you need help is a great way to identify the best people around you, because they're the ones who will either pull you up, introduce you to pull-up people, or give you the advice you need to pull yourself up.

It's scary to admit vulnerability. So we try to project the opposite, as if we can do it all ourselves. Think of how much stronger we can all be if we combine strengths, and add muscle on muscle, and skill on skill, to conquer problems that seemed bigger than any one of us alone could handle.

Need help? Just ask. If you ask for the right things, you'll be rewarded in ways you won't believe.

IT TOOK ME A WHILE TO achieve lift-off in L.A. The $3,000 I had when I moved West disappeared pretty quickly between gas money and car registration and damage deposits and rent, so I had to reach out to my friend Aaron Moore for spot loans just to scrape by.

A touchy subject, right? The very personal loan. Should you ask for one? Should you give one, if you're able?

Here's the distinction I make. For a person digging a hole— because of an addiction, or a delusion about his prospects, or an inability to get off her ass—more money is just going to vanish into the blackness down there. Hole diggers don't need money, they need to drop the shovel and get a clue, and that should be the first priority.

I like to think that Aaron could see that I wasn't just pissing away my early days in L.A. I was working as hard as I could to establish myself. The money he gave me kept me in a game that I was trying very hard to win. I was a good investment, in fact.

I took my career seriously, and I knew it wasn't going to launch itself. So, I sweated it out at Equinox constantly, and auditioned for everything Clear Talent put me up for.

I was like, "This is real life, and you better *work* at it."

I moved from class to class to class at Equinox—some, I was soaking up the instruction, some, I taught. They didn't have to ask twice if I wanted to add another class to my schedule. You know I love to teach. If this whole fitness/dance/motivation thing hadn't worked out for me: I would have been happy talking about American history or science in a high school somewhere, and seeing if I could redirect a few teenage lives.

But teaching a full schedule of classes in L.A. threw off all kinds of side benefits for me. Back benefits, booty benefits, abdominal benefits, and chest benefits.

I was building my body like a crazy person.

During those early days in L.A. I was cut. The advantage of being 24 years old, right? My testosterone was up, and I had no commitments outside the gym and the dance studio, so I was at my lifetime max as a muscle generator. I would be at the gym like 6 hours a day, no lie.

I would wake up and go teach a class.

Then, I would work out.

Then, I would add rocket fuel.

Then, I would go work out again.

Then, I would teach another class.

My life was out of balance, but that's not unusual after you make a plunge into something new. I wasn't the first one who had to prove himself by making an extraordinary effort, whether people were watching me or not. The rewards have to be personal ones, because they almost certainly won't be monetary ones, at least in the beginning.

So it pays to pick something you love to do for benefits that go beyond money, and pay off in your soul. If you can then find a way to turn a profit at it, so much the better. But at least you'll have that initial payoff for your hard work: The kind that comes directly to you, from you, rather than from somebody writing you a check.

For me, that was helping people transform their lives. For you, it might be the pleasure you take in using your math skills to make sense of a business, or your people skills to help people in an office work better with each other, or your problem solving skills to make that engine work right. It doesn't matter so much how you apply what you're good at, but rather, that you identify your unique skill in the first place.

> **TRUTHBOMB:** You're not looking for a special job, you're looking for your special gift. All that you'll give, and all that you'll get, will come from that.

As challenging as my early days in L.A. were, I was learning not only how to build my tribe, but also just how important it was. I was sharpening my skills by honing them with razor-sharp people.

Once I was standing at the front desk waiting to teach a class, and I passed the time by catching up with people, trying to put an extra charge into their day. My buddy Dale was there, listening to me, and then he comes out with it: "Shaun, you get too close to people. They're going to take over your life if you let them."

"But I *love* people," I shot back.

I was pissed off at what he said.

I didn't know any other way to behave with the people in my classes.

Any instructor can bark out exercises. That isn't why people came to me. I was just a kid at that time, but a lot of people—all ages—started showing up regularly in my classes. They would ask for help with a particular exercise or a physical problem they were having, and then those conversations would dig deeper, beyond the workout class.

It sounds like a forecast for my entire career, right?

I've thought of that exchange with Dale about a thousand times since then. He had a point: If you're giving 100 percent to the people you work with, and 100 percent to your spouse, and 100 percent to your kids, you're about 200 percent in the hole, with zero percent left to give to yourself. You're not being selfish enough if you're constantly giving and not getting the same energy back in return.

That problem comes up often with the people asking questions at a *Shaun T Live* event. A mom talks about finding time for a workout when there are so many people she needs to take care of in her life. I always say the same thing to them, but I'm directing it back at myself as well: "If you're not giving back to yourself, who will? Where's the percentage that's nurturing you, supporting your journey, helping you grow stronger? If you're not finding time for that, your clock is going to wind down."

For me, constantly delivering motivation to others is a way of reminding myself of the same values, the same steps, that have always served me well on my own path. Having the other person there is kind of a good excuse to remind myself of where I want to go and how I want to get there.

My answer to Dale, when he challenged how I relate to people, was "Whatever." Maybe I *was* out there a little too much, but then, I think that's why people kept on coming back. I was a new guy in a sometimes-hostile town. I needed to recruit support, and I never knew quite where it was going to come from.

One person it definitely came from was Pia, who worked the front desk at Equinox.

She knew I was showing up for a ton of dance auditions outside of my exercise classes, and it was working. I landed small dance gigs, and a spot on the show *Six Feet Under.* They wanted somebody to play a flirty dancer as a romantic interest. Yup, I can do that.

Even within my first 2 months in L.A., I was already setting myself apart from the dreamers and wannabes, because I was relentless.

You know RuPaul's "Lip Sync for Your Life"?

That was me, dancing during every waking hour.

Pia saw how hard I was working it, so she felt safe recommending me to her friends. One day, she said to me, "You need to meet Travis Payne."

In the dance world, that name is magic. Travis was born in Atlanta, and he busted onto the scene with a viral dance video that caught Janet Jackson's eye (just before she tied me to a table). She signed him on to her Rhythm Nation tour in 1990. That's like Jesus signing you on to a gig to walk on water with him. Travis went on to choreograph for freakin' everybody. He was working with Michael Jackson when the King of Pop moonwalked into the hereafter.

So yeah, Pia was onto something for me with Travis. I'd been in L.A. for 4 months, and I was about to meet one of the most influential figures in dance in the last 30 years.

But please believe me when I say that I was never that kind of L.A. creature who goes around meeting people based on what they could do for me. I met people because I loved them, and shared energy with them, and because I was a new guy in town. Pia was my friend before she became a useful contact, and that meant she really knew me, apart from who I was as a professional. The combination of the two made her feel comfortable turning me over to Travis.

Earlier in this chapter I encouraged you to ask for help. You should do that, definitely. But you also need to take steps to make sure you have the skills to make something of that help.

I'm thinking here of the bread that Pop-Pop handed out on

the streets of Camden. Some people ate it, got hungry again, and then came back for more. Because Pop-Pop was something of a saint, he continued to give. But he was hoping that his gift of bread would help people hear his deeper message, and join his church, and turn their lives around.

When you approach your tribe for help, do it strategically. Here's what I mean by that. If you have a work colleague who has a good relationship with the boss, it's probably useless if you simply ask her to put in a good word for you. Why should she, and for what purpose?

On the other hand, if you've noticed a breakdown in the way the office operates, talk to the people involved, study how others have solved that problem, and work to come up with a solution. Then tell your friend you just need 5 minutes of the boss's time to present the problem and the solution. It can work out for everybody: The boss gets credit for implementing your idea, your coworker gets credit for passing you and your solutions along, and you of course reap the reward for your smart thinking and hard work. Win-win-win.

TRUTHBOMB: The win always comes after the work, not as a way to avoid the work.

This ain't the lottery, where you lay out one buck to try and win a million. You want to invest the effort and build your capabilities first, then ask for help as a fuel for the rocket you're already building.

Back to my friend Pia.

She didn't just say, "Go look him up." She delivered me to him like a babe in arms. She tipped me off to an audition he was conducting, and then literally walked me up to make an introduction.

"Travis," she said. "This is Shaun. I really need for you to know him."

I danced my hardest, in part because I wanted to pay back Pia's support, but also because I always, always loved dancing more than anything.

I was in it to win it. Gave body, surrendered soul.

Then Travis walked over.

"I'm not going to pick you for this part," he said.

He had already cast the dancers who could do what I did, so I never had a chance that day.

Setback, right?

He followed up with, "Make sure you come out for my next audition, though. I'll let you know."

Oh well.

By this time, I had moved on to my second apartment in L.A., one with an actual bed. Not that I was getting a ton of sleep in it. There was just too much going on. A full schedule of classes, plus regular dance gigs.

I was barely scraping by on rent money, but I was rich in human capital. It's the best investment you can make at the beginning of any new enterprise. Meet the people who are doing what you want to do, and learn what they love about it. Immerse yourself in their stories, not just to imitate them, but to see where their passions align with yours.

That's where you make a human connection. "I love what you love," rather than, "I'd love for you to give me a huge career break."

I was very fortunate to have Pia in my circle and to have Travis Payne keeping an eye out for me. But, I wasn't lucky; I'd earned his attention with all of the hard work I'd done up to that point. That's your power connection. The work allows you to plug it in.

And wouldn't you know it, the next audition came, just as

he said it would. He was choreographing *The Ten Commandments: The Musical*, and I went on his call for dancers.

I wasn't going to be dismissed, however promisingly, this time.

I sang first, then I had to dance.

I didn't hold back one bit.

The choreography was a little different than what I was used to, but that didn't stop me.

I told them, "I can move *whatever* way."

I was dancing for my life that day, and it's no exaggeration. I *ate* it.

Ate as in gobbled it up. Spat out the bones. Went back for seconds and thirds. That audition was my gluten-free cupcake!

All done.

Travis was like, "Thank you."

That doesn't sound like a success, does it?

I was home a week later when I got a call. "You need to get down to Alley Cat Studios right away. You've been cast for the skeleton crew of *The Ten Commandments*."

That was even better than being cast for the show. I'd be part of a small group of dancers that worked closely with Travis to develop the choreography for the show, and it meant a chance to work closely with the nondancing cast.

In this case, Val Kilmer.

I wasn't star struck.

But, I was thrilled to be chosen for the group that would develop this show for the stage.

Pop-Pop! Little Shauny is dancing the Bible!

Well, maybe it wouldn't have been his favorite version, seeing as this was a pre-Broadway tryout. And our outfits were pretty skimpy. Not exactly the Mormon Tabernacle Choir up there.

But, I was so happy to make the show. Then, it hit me, in the pit of my stomach: *Oh my God. I made the show!*

Now what?

I wasn't a classically trained dancer. I never took a technique class. I knew modern and hip hop and a little bit of jazz, but this was like a street-ball guy suiting up for the NBA. The game was *faster*.

Yes, I had an aptitude for it, I had energy for it, and I could sell my moves to an audience. But, could I sell them to this room full of dance pros? People who were hooked in with Janet Jackson? Britney Spears?

It was another perfect opportunity for Shaun T to fail, or to break through. Amazing and uncomfortable at the same time.

TRUTHBOMB: To raise your game, raise the level of the people you're playing with.

I walked into the rehearsal room and thought, I don't know *anybody*. And this wasn't like dance class in New Jersey, where you learn it step-by-step. In this crowd, there was literally no time to mess up, or I would have been back out the door just as quickly as I had walked in.

Travis was like, "Okay, here's the step."

Boom.

"Turn here."

Boom boom.

"Grab the girl. Lift."

Boom boom *boom*.

"Now, with the music."

We'd do it that way once while Travis watched, chin in hand, thinking it over.

"No wait, reverse the steps. One and two and three and *go!*"

It was never the same. I'd be turning to the dancer next to me: "*What* did he just say?"

Fortunately, the woman I asked would turn out to be my

friend Tania, who would eventually go through the DVD wars with me, from *Hip Hop Abs* all the way to *CIZE*.

When I first reached out, she might have been a stranger who would have stepped over my body if I collapsed on that dance floor. Instead, she reached back. The miracle of admitting I was vulnerable!

Tania supported me that first day, and we ended up supporting each other in everything we did for the next two decades. With help from Tania and too many others to count, I moved from gym ratting at Rowan to getting biblical at the Kodak (now Dolby) Theater in L.A.—home of the Oscars and, for the 6-week run of *The Ten Commandments*, Shaun T.

I hadn't "made it." I wasn't dancing in the end zone by any means. But, I was working with and learning from incredible people. And, I was still dancing, and that was a dream in itself.

Here's the lesson in all of this. It isn't that Shaun made a bunch of friends who furthered his career. Rather, it's that you have the ability to look past the limitations of your current circle, especially if it's so small that it's squeezing you into an uncomfortable space, or holding you back from rising higher.

Make connections, and give people reasons to connect with you. The stronger you are, the stronger your circle is, and the more you can all accomplish. Together.

Who's your Pia? And will she want to introduce you to your Travis? Get to work, and they'll find you.

Appearing on stage in L.A. in *The Ten Commandments* was the culmination of all the hard work I'd done as a dancer, and it introduced me to an amazing group of friends and mentors. But, it also started me thinking about my own rules for living. Ten is a good number! With apologies to Pop-Pop, let me take a couple of tablets from God's own playbook, and hand down my own Ten TransformaShaun Commandments on how to go biblical with your own success.

Thou shalt forget about "instant success"

Calling successes instant *anything* ignores the million individual steps required along the way. If you miss even one of those steps, you might trip coming through the doorway, or more likely, not make it there at all. When you're looking for your breakthrough, remember that it will be a product of a long investment of time (remember the 10,000 hours?), skills (uniquely yours), and effort (see Commandment #2). Better start now.

COMMANDMENT #2:
Thou shalt honor thy passions

If you're going to be in it for the long haul, you better have a hot fire in your engine. Passion, fascination, curiosity, commitment is your fire. What fuels yours? Each of us has a unique gift that we can develop with the right care and attention. Start by asking yourself: What is it that you do not because it's next on your to-do list, but because nobody could stop you from doing it if they tried? Building a world-class skill takes world-class effort. Start with what you're willing to work hard at, and see where that can take you.

COMMANDMENT #3:
Thou shalt build thy foundation

Your passion won't mean a thing if you don't practice the skills that will help you translate it into action. Let your passion lead you through a deep exploration of the subject and all the ways it's expressed in the world. It means that you'll be learning new skills, and need to practice, practice, and practice them some more. If it's truly your passion, the fire will burn through rounds of confusion and discomfort until you can develop your expertise in a way that's uniquely yours.

COMMANDMENT #4:
Thou shalt not covet thy neighbor's success

Here's a big pitfall. Looking around too much at what others have done can cause you to miss what *you're* meant to do. You can learn a lot by looking side to side to see what others are up to, but not if you let it divert you off your own path. Develop who *you* are and what *you* can do.

COMMANDMENT #5:
Thou shalt carefully recruit thy posse

Dale, the guy who questioned the energy I gave to my students at Equinox, was probably right. I didn't need to be so friendly. And yet, my people skills helped me get many of my biggest breaks. By taking a genuine interest in people, I was able to make real connections that led to them wanting to help me. Jobs are a mix of the personal and the professional, and you'll be judged on both of them. So, work hard at both.

COMMANDMENT #6:
Thou shalt not expect perfection

You heard me bashing the pursuit of perfection a lot in this book. In fact, your desire to get things *exactly* right could keep you from moving forward at all. Perfectionists tend to be super-self-critical, and they can get hung up on small details that don't matter in the long run. I'm not saying that details aren't important, but they're not the only thing that matters. Cut yourself some slack on perfection, and keep your eyes on the bigger prize, whatever it may be. Perfection happens for a moment, but change is constant. Open yourself up to change, and master that.

COMMANDMENT #7:
Thou shalt honor thy small successes

I'll say it again: Fit is just a number. The milestones that are important are the ones where you realize that you feel better, or are getting better, or are surprising yourself with how deep you can dig. And, those are the moments that you should celebrate—every day, if possible! It just reminds me that our journeys in life aren't usually made up of giant leaps. They're an accumulation of small steps in the right direction. Even small steps in the wrong direction teach you something. If we really want to make progress in life, we need to celebrate each of those small steps, because they're what get you places. If you have a long way to go, stop looking at the horizon. Start looking at an achievable distance nearby, and do everything you can to get there. Then, celebrate (briefly)!

COMMANDMENT #8:
Thou shalt put the haters in their place

This is the flip side of Commandment #5, where you gather your posse. Because, just as surely as you need goals to keep your life moving forward, you'll attract people who will delight in telling you that you'll never get there. But there's a difference between people who tell you you're hopeless, and people who help you strategize the steps along a difficult journey. Figure out who's merely pointing out hurdles, and who's helping you develop the stride to jump over them.

Thou shalt reset the GPS when you need to

It's okay for your goal to change. That's the thrill of the journey, right? You'll have a different perspective 3 miles down the road than you do when you're just starting out, and that's a good thing. If you set your sights on traveling from Jersey to L.A., and find out that Kansas City is where you were meant to be, that's an amazing result. Plus, the barbecue is really good there. You may never reach your original destination, but that's not the point, anyway. You're constantly moving, and you'll often surprise yourself with the arrival point. "Recalculating" just might be the most thrilling words you can hear from your internal GPS.

Thou shalt be willing to leave thy old life behind

I put this last, but maybe it should have been first. Really, it's a kind of subtext to every commandment here. We so often prefer where we are—no matter how difficult or annoying or just plain *boring* it is—to the unknown ahead. But sometimes, the devil you know literally *is* a devil. In order to move on, you need to believe in a better place and trust yourself to reach it. At the start, it takes imagination, but soon you can fill it up with the details and skills that make it your new reality. And that devil? He's shrinking in the rearview mirror.

T IS FOR TRANSFORMATION

SUPERPOWER #2: FULL OUT-EDNESS

Full out confidence means that you believe in your ability to handle anything that comes down the street. There is situational confidence ("I know I can finish this workout/learn this dance move/write this book") and general self-confidence ("I can hit life's serves, lobs, volleys, and move past the errors"). Full-out people believe they can make any situation work for them. They live to see a *new* day, not Groundhog Day. The downside: Overdoing full out-edness can lead to a cocky, know-it-all attitude, so when friends tell you how crazy you're being, you won't even hear them.

SELF-TEST:
ARE YOU GOING FULL OUT?

[1 = That's me! 6 = That's totally not me!]

1. I don't second-guess myself.

| 1 | 2 | 3 | 4 | 5 | 6 |

2. I can make any situation work out.

| 1 | 2 | 3 | 4 | 5 | 6 |

3. If life gives me lemons (or even limes), I make margaritas.

| 1 | 2 | 3 | 4 | 5 | 6 |

4. I focus on my strengths. (What weaknesses?)

| 1 | 2 | 3 | 4 | 5 | 6 |

5. I believe in my abilities.

| 1 | 2 | 3 | 4 | 5 | 6 |

SCORE BOX

Mostly 1s and 2s: Like a toddler on Mountain Dew.

Mostly 3s and 4s: On the cusp. Still limiting yourself, though.

Mostly 5s and 6s: Still in the starting blocks. Let yourself go!

SHAUN T'S
CONFIDENCE-BUILDERS

EXERCISE #1

Strike the Superwoman (or Superman) pose. Amy Cuddy—search YouTube for her Ted Talk "Your Body Language Shapes Who You Are"—was right: You can fake it until you *become* it. Impersonating Superwoman changes your posture *and* your life. Stand tall! Chest out! Head up! Leap buildings! Be super! Okay, it's just an act, but the act becomes *you,* if you stick with it.

EXERCISE #2

Change your soundtrack. Remember what I was saying about the life soundtrack? It's the stream of words that we use to describe ourselves to ourselves. Let's face it, that record would probably have a warning label: CAUTION: LYRICS CONTAIN VIOLENT IMAGES, PROFANITY, AND OTHER STUFF NOT SUITABLE FOR HAPPY PEOPLE. Listen to how you address yourself, inside. If it's "You f*&^%g idiot!", change your soundtrack to something more accepting, supportive, and inspirational. Save the curses for your enemies; reserve the best for yourself.

EXERCISE #3

Invest in exteriors. I'm not just talking about a better haircut or new clothes. Though I'm also not ruling them out. When I was trying to make it in L.A. I gladly went to Ross for last year's styles at used-clothing prices. People buy how you present yourself, and you can do that for free by maintaining eye contact; by speaking slow, loud, and clear; and by smiling more. You'll come off as confident, and people will believe in you more. That should lead to even more smiling.

EXERCISE #4

SWOT the difference. Pull out a piece of paper and list your:

Strengths: What unique skills, knowledge, insight, or passion do you bring to the world?

Weaknesses: Be honest now. What do you hate doing, or repeatedly fail at? Is an addiction starting to mess up your home and work life?

Opportunities: Your supervisor announced that she's leaving the company? Your neighbor is looking for a partner in a business venture? Your online sales initiative is taking off?

Threats: Is your new boss skeptical of your skills? Is your business in a down cycle?

If you're taking this exercise seriously, you will have filled four pages with your strengths, weaknesses, opportunities, and threats. As you scan them, look for themes that emerge. How do your strengths match the threats? Which weaknesses can you bolster to take advantage of your opportunities? And which of these themes is ultimately going to be most important to you, and provide the most opportunities for growth? Distill those down into three or four specific goals—I'll boost my opportunities by doing X, I'll handle threat Y by developing personal strength Z, I'll take class W to bolster weakness V. Organize your personal to-do list around those goals. Doing the work to figure out not only what's holding you back but also what can drive you forward can give you reason to *really* believe, and take you there.

EXERCISE #5
Distance yourself from Debbie Downer. You know this lady. When the sun pops up, she finds a reason to criticize it. And you. And that new skirt you're wearing. So, as extra credit for the exercise at the end of Chapter Eight, draw up a list of the five most negative people you know, and a separate list of the five most positive. Now draw up a life path that puts you among the positives, and limits access to the negatives. Changing up the soundtrack of what you're hearing all day can change your mental direction at the speed of sound. And, don't forget: Maybe a quick word with Debbie Downer could change her tune as well.

EXERCISE #6
Put it on the line. Your greatest fear is public speaking? Teach a class in a subject you know cold. Embarrassed by your body? Wear spandex to your new exercise class. Think your opinions aren't worth listening to? Join the book club at your public library. Your demons shrink when you shine a light on them. The bigger they seem, the more reps you need to make them disappear. So, get started. Now. What's your first action?

EXERCISE #7
Switch it up. It can, in fact, be dangerous to exercise to exhaustion. But, the opposite extreme has its downsides

as well. It can simply be a waste of time to do the same exercise routine every day, with the same amount of effort, until death do you part. So I'm going to throw down a challenge at you: Within your workouts, you should constantly be switching up the amount of weight you're using, the number of reps you're doing, or your exertion level while you're doing it. That's one of the reasons I've included three workout routines in the Appendix on page 252. If you're new to Shaun T world, any of them can shock your system into a new mode of fitness, just like I did with the workers at the PSERG nuclear power plant in Jersey. Same with you: If you're not turning up the juice in your efforts, your fitness levels go into brownout.

Can You Go <u>Too</u> Full Out?

Stop bragging in your Facebook posts, and . . .

- Join groups of people who can teach you something.

- Learn a new skill in an area where you're entirely ignorant. Kick-ass accountant? Take a cooking class. Made of muscle? Let me see you coordinate that with timing and grace in *CIZE*, or hone it through tennis lessons.

- Tackle a problem that's bigger than you are, like hunger in your neighborhood, or illiteracy in city schools. Remind yourself of all you've been given, and start sharing the wealth.

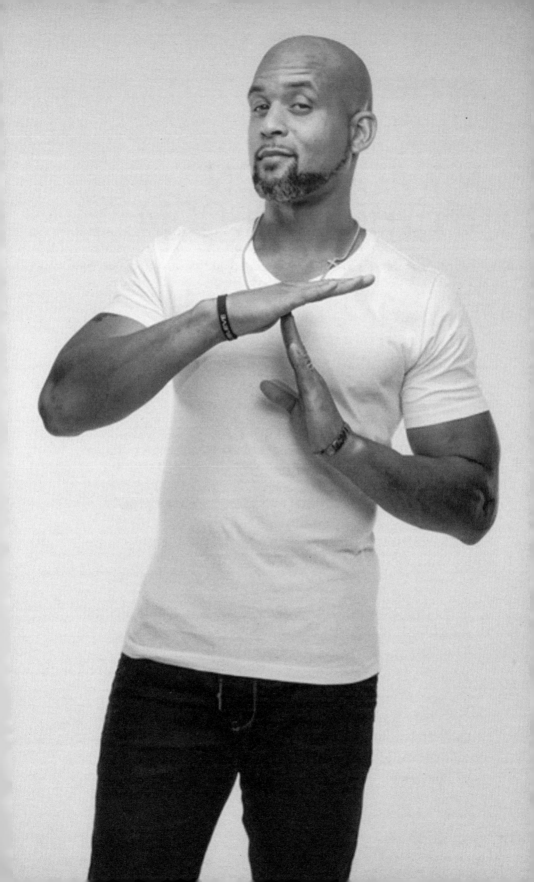

CHAPTER ELEVEN

MY AUDITION IN THE BEDROOM

Maybe you feel like you're stuck with certain chapters in your life story that you wish you could go back and rewrite. Maybe you're investing a lot more energy than you realize into maintaining a situation that you're not happy with, when you could be diverting that energy as a force for change.

> **TRUTHBOMB:** Today isn't over, and tomorrow hasn't happened yet. That's the great thing about both of them. You create them with your actions.

Likewise with that circle around you. People can be quicksand, sucking you under. But, they can also be your trampoline, launching you back up when you're heading down. And, the degree to which they do one or the other depends on which ones you seek out, and which ones you close out.

So, your book isn't written yet, and your story isn't over. Maybe the early chapters make you cringe when you read them. But, as long as you're still living, you can direct the story wherever you want it to go.

Don't let anybody else write those chapters or dictate the plot to you. Take charge of them. *You* are the author. Write your story. Make the surprise ending one you'll celebrate for the rest of your life.

YOU COULD LOOK AT MY CAREER and think right place, right time. Shaun T was just lucky to end up in that fitness club, in that audition, in that job.

Or, you could look at it the way I do. I left the home where I was abused, left my comfort zone in New Jersey, slept on my mattress with a hole in it, and still operated with full energy on my seven (or more?) jobs in L.A.

You know where my story stands today, so it's easy to overlook the choices that I made to bring me here. I was fighting through it day by day, at times confused, disappointed, tempted, lonely, tired—just like you. But, I was also as energized, excited, grateful, and outgoing as I could be.

My story seems inevitable now. Yours probably does to you, too. Both are the result of a series of decisions. At any moment, you can change the decisions and commit to those changes, and then your results will change, too.

I'm not saying that any of it is easy. I am saying that it's all up to you.

I WAS RUNNING WITH SOME COOL people in L.A. But, I never forgot what it was like to grow up poor in Philly and Jersey. In some sense I never stopped being that little kid, holding tight onto that quarter my mom gave me to buy some juice when I got to school.

That street sense stuck with me all the way out to L.A., and even beyond. Scott is one of the calmest people you'll ever meet, so when we get into a tough spot, he's always saying, "Let's think this through before we react."

But, I'm still thinking: *I'm gonna fight back before they get my juice money!*

So, you can see my motivation when I arrived in L.A.: I didn't even *have* juice money! I booked as many dance gigs as I could, while teaching a full load of classes. I always had the sense that I was just a sprained ankle away from being broke at any moment. So, I worked like each job might be all that kept me off the street.

That last-quarter mentality is a genius motivator. I still live that way today, because it works.

Counting quarters helped me sidestep the L.A. traps lots of newcomers fall into. A lot of them confused the distractions of L.A. life—the cars, the clothes, the parties, the celebs—with the means to success. They thought that if you dressed well enough, had a sweet ride, went to enough parties, and sucked up to the right people, you'd have an inside track to the high lifestyle.

My take was that talking to drunks, looking fly, and driving something you'd worry about parking in the street, is not the ticket to anything but an empty bank account. The Beverly Center, the Auto Gallery, and the Polo Lounge do a lot of economic damage to people who are more hopeful than hard-working.

My approach? Focus on what you're doing, rather than how you look doing it.

In fact, I believe that's the secret to every bit of success I've had.

Remember the first fitness class I taught at Rowan? I succeeded there not because I looked cute with a little sweat on me. It was because I cared about every person who walked into that room to exercise that day. I saw individuals on a journey just like mine, and tailored the workout for each of them. It came from inside me and worked inside each of them.

Same was true, only amplified, by the time I started teaching fitness classes in L.A. I had taught hundreds of classes by that time, encountered thousands of personal stories of the people in my classes, and I learned something very important: No two stories are alike. No two needs are the same. I respected all of them. I was a teacher because I needed to learn, too.

The only things I cared about were: Did I perform well in the audition? Did I serve the needs of my class? I wanted to be known for who I was internally, not what basketball shorts and tank top I was wearing. And that couldn't distract anybody from who I really was, underneath it all.

Even today, people are always telling me: "You need to be at this party . . . meet these people . . . be in this room."

Hardly.

TRUTHBOMB: When you go for a new opportunity, showcase *what you can do,* instead of who you know or how you look.

If I was true to my own experience and believed in the work I had done, something interesting was going to come of it.

Here are a few questions for you.

Have you found the real you?

Have you worked hard enough to make people notice?

Do they respect the *real* you well enough to pass you along to the people they respect the most?

Have you had it with these questions?

Okay, I'll stop.

Just want to make sure that you're seeing the connection between my story and your own opportunities for transformation. After all, that's the name of the game (and of this book).

It takes years of intricate planning to build a DVD (or streaming) exercise program that will actually help people.

You need to develop a concept for the program, put moves together, recruit trainers and a test panel of exercisers, and make sure that it's going to work for people before you even think about turning on the cameras.

It just so happened that Kathy Smith, an exercise innovator and goddess of the highest order, was looking for instructors to help run her test group for her next video. A pal of mine at Equinox knew her, thought of me, and said, "I can introduce you."

Her address was in Brentwood, in L.A. I drove Focusina up to the curb, killed the blaring car stereo, and stepped into the street—baseball cap on, pants slung low, tank top, little MapQuest printout (remember them?) in hand.

And yet, I had the full 10,000 hours backing me up: as a dancer, as a workout leader, as a guy who knew how to motivate change in people's lives, including my own. So, I felt pretty confident as I rolled up her sidewalk. Opportunity doesn't always knock . . . sometimes there's a doorbell. I pressed the button, and a pretty blonde lady swung the door open. Kathy Smith took my big paw in her iron-lady grip, and said, "You're Shaun?"

Kathy Smith practically invented video exercise in the 1980s (okay, Jane Fonda, too). She'd had a string of successes spanning two decades by the time I met her. I wasn't even thinking of doing my own DVDs at this point. I just wanted another paying job to put gas in Focusina, and she had a job to offer: Leading test groups for her new program *Project You*.

Enter Shaun T, who had spent years running the gym rat maze.

Kathy Smith taught and motivated people all across the country, and just watching her showed me how to expand my world. I needed to move beyond just Shaun—hustling for a living, gig by gig, person to person, in L.A.—to a bigger pool of people who needed help.

"I'm running a test group," she told me that morning at her house. "I need somebody who can teach and is really energetic."

The only question: What kind of energy was she looking for?

We were on the same mission: To connect with people, and give them a hand up. Or, better still, to give them ways *to lift themselves up.*

But, she still had to put me to the test.

"Let's go upstairs to my bedroom," she said. "It's lined with mirrors. You want to play around a little bit? Make up some routines?"

Play around? Routines? Mirrors?

Damn.

I have never mounted stairs quite the way I did to her bedroom that day.

"What if she hits on me?" I asked myself. "What am I going to do?" What kind of audition *is* this?

A small, shriveled voice spoke up from down below, in my shorts: "I don't care how pretty she is! I ain't doing *nothing.*"

We arrived in her bedroom, surrounded by mirrors as advertised. She said: "Let's work out!"

I could do *that!*

Who was I kidding? She probably knew I was gay, and anyway, she wanted to use my body in other ways. Like, you know, professionally. Ha!

We had a ball. Threw out exercises, motivated ourselves and each other. It was clear that we shared a vision for our workouts and a mission to help people. She immediately signed me on to lead the test group for her next workout program. She was a pioneer in the leotard-and-headband school of fitness, incorporating music and movement into routines for a suburban crowd. It wasn't exactly Philly-style, but it was hugely popular, and I felt so lucky to be a part of it. Soon, my already packed days were even more packed. You know the traffic in L.A. If you leave at 5:55 a.m., the drive (anywhere) takes 15 minutes. If you leave at 6:00 a.m., you're in traffic for an hour, or you may never get there (anywhere).

So, Shaun was popping out of bed and onto the road at 5:45 a.m.—gotta be professional, people—and in the lot at Kathy's workout space around 6:00, where I'd recline my seat in Focusina and finish my night's sleep. Then, up at 6:50 and into the studio by 7:00 to welcome my first test group participants.

I'd do the same thing every afternoon. I shuffled that around my 10 other fitness classes and regular dance gigs.

Not the most convenient schedule, you say? Listen up:

TRUTHBOMB: When you're doing what you love, you'll wake up at any time and drive anywhere to do it.

When you've found your passion, obstacles—even L.A. traffic jams—melt before it.

The best part of those classes were Kathy's students—largely comprised of people who were unhappy with the extra pounds they had put on. I was energetic alright, because they deserved my best effort. And, when it came time for the student evaluations, the payoff was real. It was measured in waistlines shrunk and lives changed, and they raved about Team Kathy-Shaun. Here's the funny thing, of course: They were thanking us for something *they did themselves.*

Kathy had a couple of assistants working at her home office, managing her businesses and her appearance schedule. That allowed her to be home with her daughters, dividing attention between them and her work. She even invited me to a few of their school events, to do fitness demonstrations and lead workouts. I guess that worked out okay, because one of her daughters—Kate Grace—sprinted into the Rio Olympics in 2016.

Good job, Mom.

The lesson here isn't that you should find somebody successful and leech off them. Instead, it's to conduct yourself as a professional, build valuable skills, and constantly work with the best people you can find. If that means you're a little restless in your career, that's the way it is. As long as you do your part, find the way you can make a real contribution, the best will seek you out, just like Kathy did for me.

Her most surprising gift to me wasn't even the test group or her professional organization. She fixed my teeth.

I had no dental insurance at the time, and no intention to smile at a dental hygienist. But, I was in pain, and one day I mentioned it after class.

Some health example I was, right?

Kathy marched me down to her dentist, got my aching teeth treated, and paid the bill. I've had reason to smile about her ever since.

That's full-service mentorship, right?

That's what happens when you choose your Five well!

DEALING WITH TRAFFIC WAS NEVER MY favorite part of life in L.A., but it did give me time to think, as I inched along the 405 Freeway, along with everybody else in California.

And maybe, because of that, I tend to build roadmaps from the present to where I want to end up.

Here's how it works.

First, spend some time looking in the rearview mirror, identifying every right turn, every wrong turn, every crash, every time you got lost, everyone who gave you good directions, and all the people who sent you off a cliff as well. (I hope you did the exercise on page 55. If not, why not? Get back there!) This is a no-blame, no-shame activity—it's only about learning how to recognize how you ended up on a path that you didn't like. Once you figure out the route that got you where you are today, start thinking about whether there were any common road signs. What kinds of things are going on in your life around the time you start reaching for the whole carton of ice cream? What kinds of feelings do you have around a person who genuinely has your back? The more you review the turns and detours that take you on healthy or negative paths, the better you will be at recognizing them on the road ahead of you.

That's how you make your windshield bigger than the rearview mirror.

Going forward, you'll be able to spot familiar potholes and remember the blind curves, and avoid them. You'll recognize the ditch you drove into that one time. The place where your battery went dead from leaving that dome light on. The DUI you earned from lack of self-control with the corkscrew. The time you sat waiting by that curb forever waiting for a tow.

When you know the familiar road hazards in your life, you can hit the brakes, swerve, or change lanes whenever necessary. You spend less time wandering lost and more time accelerating to your destination.

I know I'm making it sound easy, but I've lived through the same struggle, and I sympathize with both of us. But, if you do the work to figure out how you got here, you really can pull off your transformation going forward, and make it stick.

TRUTHBOMB: If you understand your wrong turns, then you'll know how to keep your nose pointed toward your destination from now on.

That doesn't mean that you're done driving, or that any single destination is the end of your road. Life is the ultimate point-to-point-to-point journey. You make a series of turns, and then the view starts to change, and, suddenly, you find you can reach new places from there. Or, that you're headed for a crash.

And I learned all that while waiting in traffic! Make good use of your time, even the annoying parts!

THINGS WERE GOING SO WELL FOR me in L.A. that I started to tell myself, "I'm locked and loaded, here."

I was the most physically fit I'd ever been in my life.

I was 27 years old, and I felt amazing.

I was on the top of the world, dancing, living. I wasn't on cloud 9. More like cloud 10.5.

Too bad I nearly died right about then.

I nearly did.

Just after *Commandments* wrapped, and as I was beginning my relationship with Kathy, I'd been cast in a production of *Pippin*. During the first week of the show, I got a stomachache. Not a too-much-candy stomachache. More like a the-world-is-about-to-end stomachache. But, like I told you, I was a professional, and I was doing what I loved: dancing. You don't dance with your stomach (unless you're a belly dancer), so I said: The show must go on.

But, the pain kept getting worse. My belly felt like a fireball, then a supernova. I had to go to the bathroom all the time, but when I would unholster and release my bladder . . . nothing.

After a couple of days, I finally decided that I couldn't white-knuckle my way through the pain anymore. But, instead of calling 911, I took a shower and put on some nice sweats. I wanted to look good for my drive to the hospital!

If you take nothing else from this book, take this: Pick up the damn phone and call for help if you're about to die, okay?

I jumped into Focusina, and, despite the fact that I could barely see the road through my pain, I drove toward the nearest hospital. I soon realized that I'd never make it, but then I spotted an Urgent Care center. I pointed the car at it.

I told the triage nurse, "I need help right now. My stomach is about to explode."

A doctor rushed in.

He took one look at me—fit guy! big pain!—and started feeling around for a hernia. I told him that I lifted female dancers into the air for a living, but that I did it with good form. So, probably no hernia. Best possible explanation out of the way. Onto the worst.

"It's either a hernia, or your appendix ruptured," he said. "Get this guy into an ambulance!"

In the E.R., they sent me in for x-rays, but nobody found the reason for the pain, and it was immense. They set me up with my own private morphine drip, and I hit that button, hard.

It hit right back and spilled my guts with the most wrenching vomiting I hope I'll ever do in my life. You've seen *The Exorcist?* Yeah, a full-on Linda Blair.

Three days later a doctor came in, looked me over, and said, "I think you have AIDS," based on absolutely nothing.

When you've spent 3 days having your intestines pulled out through your bellybutton, you'd welcome *any* explanation, if it would stop the pain.

But, I wasn't having unprotected sex, and I wasn't a drug user, so I didn't go with that AIDS idea. I was like, "No. Next diagnosis."

They signed me up for surgery. But, I wasn't nervous. Have you ever been so sick that you thought: *If I die right now, I'm mad cool with that. Bye Felicia!* Bring on the gas, boys, and don't wake me up unless you fix it.

When I came to, I was on a gurney rolling down a corridor in the hospital. I was groggy, but I could already sense that something important was missing.

Oh, right. The pain! Gone! (Temporarily, it turned out.)

Still, I was overwhelmed, like, what was *wrong* with me?

Eventually, my surgeon showed up, and the answers finally came.

"Your appendix ruptured," he told me.

Right, like the guy at Urgent Care said. Could have saved me a couple days of crazy hurt, doc!

"It was hidden behind your intestines; that's why we couldn't see it. If we'd waited another day, you would have died from the poisons it released when it blew."

I sneaked a look at the small, vertical scar under my belly button. It didn't seem like much of a cut for such a big pain in the gut.

"I was going to cut you from down here all the way up to the top of your sternum to open you up," he told me. "But when I looked at your abs, I thought, 'I'm not messing that up.'"

Another reason to stay fit, right?

And, when you think that my first break in fitness videos would be *Hip Hop Abs*, that doctor saved my body for a career move I didn't know I'd be making.

I thanked the doctor for sparing my abdomen, but then he hit me with a punch in the gut: "Your recovery is going to be harder because I had to go in through such a small space to clean you out. The sooner you get up and start moving, the better your recovery will be."

That's where my life lesson came in.

I knew I had to get moving, so I had them hook my IV into a wheeled cart, and I had a friend bring in headphones. It was way too painful for me to walk much, but here's the beauty part: I found I could dance.

So, I went with that.

First, I moved one arm. Then, the other.

One foot, then two feet.

My legs.

My body.

Ever so carefully, one move at a time, music became my painkiller, and dance was my physical therapist. I found a quiet hallway, flooded my brain with rhythm, and hip hopped with my IV trolley.

The pain didn't stand a chance once I could dance.

TRUTHBOMB: Let the things that you love help carry you past the stuff you hate.

I'm not telling you to ignore doctor's orders, of course. But, I am saying that there will be painful moments on your journey where you have to muster all your will to make another step forward. That's where you tap into the thing that motivates you the most, that you enjoy the most, and the one that's at the heart of who you are and what you want to become.

For me, it was dance. For you, it could be your skill with numbers or your visual sense or your talent for making connections with people. Whatever your bedrock ability is, rely on it to carry you past the pain into your promised land. It won't make the journey any shorter or less painful, but it will help you sustain your effort as you move forward.

Always forward.

T IS FOR TRANSFORMATION

SUPERPOWER #3: CREATIVITY

When resourceful people are in a tough spot, they MacGyver it into a sweet spot. They can brainstorm lots of paths to a goal, and they tap unusual people for help. They Google and YouTube away until they're experts. They look for new ways to solve old problems, and old ways to solve new ones. Creativity means that you're never stuck, because you're always inventing ways to keep moving forward. But, it's also possible to be *too* resourceful, overlooking obvious solutions and creating more work than is necessary.

SELF-TEST:
HOW CREATIVE ARE YOU?

[1 = That's me! 6 = That's totally not me!]

1. If it's broken, I fix it.

1	2	3	4	5	6

2. When I'm stuck, I wiggle out of it.

1	2	3	4	5	6

3. When other people are stuck, they holla for me.

1	2	3	4	5	6

4. When I hit a hurdle, I go over, around, under, or through it.

1	2	3	4	5	6

5. I look under rocks, on the top shelf, or over the rainbow for solutions.

1	2	3	4	5	6

SCORE BOX

Mostly 1s and 2s: You're the handyman or handywoman.

Mostly 3s and 4s: You could use a few more tools in the box.

Mostly 5s and 6s: You need to replace a burned-out idea bulb.

SHAUN T'S
CREATIVITY WORKOUT

EXERCISE #1: Know where to go

Enroll in the University of YouTube. If you need to know how to do it, somebody has posted a video to explain it to you. Concentrate on the ones with the most likes and views, and you can become your own handyman or -woman.

Get to know Ted Talks. Sometimes, you need to go beyond how to replace a washer in the faucet and find out how to fix a relationship, or how to project more confidence at the office. Ted Talks present life mojo in 10- to 20-minute seminars, and they can transform relationships. Press play on Jenna McCarthy's "What You Don't Know About Marriage" if you don't believe me.

EXERCISE #2: Build your confidence

- **Help others solve their problems.** Be a volunteer counselor in your area of expertise, or simply pitch in with friends and relatives. The more problems you help solve, the more you'll see yourself as someone who invents solutions and gets sh*t done.

- **Organize your tools.** The messes in your life (kitchen, office, car trunk, garage, attic, workbench) communicate a message loud and clear—you can't handle stuff. Control your chaos! Make sure help is handy!

- **Go for a run, swim laps, take a walk.** The repetitive motion in exercise fires up your brain synapses, making electrical hook-ups between brain regions that just wouldn't happen if you were sitting in a chair in your office. If you need a brainstorm, start a sweat storm. The two are often connected.

- **Take a long, hot shower afterward.** I get a lot of my best ideas in the shower, for two reasons: (1) I take one in the morning, when my mind is rested, and I scan the day ahead for problems and solutions. That's a perfect moment for creative thinking. (2) In the shower, there's usually nothing else going on. No e-mails to answer, no tweets to retweet. And you'd better not be using Instagram in there. In the absence of other stimulation, you're trapped inside your own head. But, that means you're free to let your mind roam for 6 to 7 minutes. Or 15, like me. It's amazing how much you can process in that amount of time. Just don't forget your great ideas while you towel off!

Are You **Too** Creative?

- **Avoid immobility.** Are you the sort of person who spends so much time assembling the tools that you never start the job? Do you come up with a good idea and then spend most of your time finding reasons not to follow through on it? Simply start. You'll develop momentum once you shift the car out of neutral. Or reverse.

- **Limit the inputs.** Everybody has an opinion, but that doesn't mean that you have to listen to all of them. Recruit a mentor, listen hard, and shut out the noise. You'll have enough on your mind without inviting competing voices into your head. Focus your research, and move forward.

- **KISS it.** *K*eep *I*t *S*imple, *S*weetheart. If your head is buzzing with a thousand details, none of them will get the attention they need. Be ruthless with your priority list, and progress is at hand.

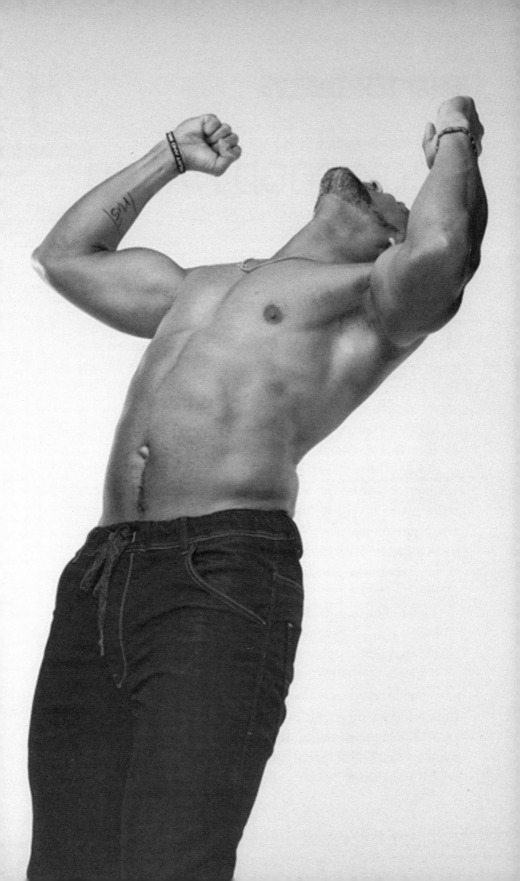

CHAPTER TWELVE

LOOK GOOD NAKED

This may be the most difficult thing I've asked you to do yet: Take off your clothes, step in front of the mirror, and do an inventory. What looks good to you? What do you dislike? Where do your eyes go first? What embarrasses you most? What's your worst quality? Your best?

I know what you're thinking: Easy for me to direct you to do all that. I work out for a living, after all.

But I'm the guy who gained a bunch of weight really quickly, stretching the skin on his waist, his butt, under his arms, above his chest. I have actually been relaxing on a beach when somebody asks, "What are those scars from? Did you have surgery? Were you on steroids?"

I tell them the truth: "They're from when I gained a lot of weight really fast."

And, I'm okay with that.

Every scar and every imperfection that I have on my body, I embrace now.

It hasn't always been that way. At a different point in my life, I used to avoid getting naked in the locker room and in theater changing rooms because of those stretch marks. Now, I'm like, "If I never gained that weight and produced those scars, I would have never had the chance to dig deep to get where I am today."

You don't have to live up to some ideal. That's only possible on a magazine cover, with a digital artist wiping the blemishes off the photograph, and pumping up the muscle. It's one of the reasons I love my *Men's Health* magazine cover shot from January 2015. It shows the scar from my appendix surgery!

TRUTHBOMB: Every wrinkle, blemish, and gray hair marks a step on your journey, so accept them as you accept yourself.

Love the journey.

Love the road signs.

Love the traveler (you!).

Your success point is when you can look at yourself naked, accept the imperfections, and see your beauty.

Don't compare yourself to any other person, because the moment you do that, other obnoxious questions pop up: Is she sexier than I am? Does she have a better ass?

In fact, "she" doesn't matter.

You do.

You're all you'll ever have.

The real you.

The naked you.

That's the person you need to accept.

Say it to yourself: "I am amazing as who I am today."

Shaun T hears you and agrees!

OK. Put your clothes back on. Well done, you!

I KNOW WHAT I'M TALKING ABOUT, in regard to nakedness. At one point, I was a professional at it.

At about the same time I was showing a lot of skin as a singing-dancing slave in *The Ten Commandments*, I began my well-paid career as a stripper.

I attribute that positive career turn to my professionalism.

Creative fields are populated by creative people, and they also tend to be creative with their time—stay up until dawn, sleep until noon.

But, I was never that guy.

I valued my work too much to leave anything to chance, even when that work involved removing my clothes and dancing.

Stop me if you've heard this one before: I made the connection to stripping through someone I met on another job. One day after class, I got to talking with a woman in my Kathy Smith test group. We had already bonded by sweating together, so I asked her what she did for a living.

"My husband and I manage the Crow Bar," she told me.

I tried not to let my mouth gape open in surprise. She was talking about one of L.A.'s most famous, wildest, most notorious gay clubs, back in the day, and one of the things they were famous/notorious for were their dancers. And, okay, I'd been a few times, and, yes, I'd wondered about the men dancing in those boy boxes. It didn't look like hard labor. The people in the club weren't exactly showing up to critique the technical skills of the dancers in G-strings.

I asked my new friend how much the dancers made.

"Six hundred dollars per night in tips, and they can enjoy the club for free."

Los Angeles: The land of opportunity.

I didn't include a line about stripping on my résumé, but I did have some experience from back home. Atlantic City required dancers with lots of different skills, including gyration in a G-string. If I danced as a giant mouse, I could certainly dance as myself, in my own skin.

My friend Aaron used to drive over there with me to keep me company and to collect my cast-off clothing, so he was there when I was called into a bachelorette party. I aimed to please, and my customers were certainly enthusiastic. I can still remember Aaron shouting with glee and greed, "Girl, we need to grab these twenties raining down on the floor!"

If the customers weren't too proud to toss them at me or tuck them into my G-string, I wasn't too proud to accept them with full gratitude.

Soon after my conversation with Kathy Smith's student, I made my debut at the Crow Bar. I danced a few nights a week, showing up (and off) on time, giving good value, conducting myself as a professional, and pocketing tips for my trouble and exposure.

Are you shocked that your motivation mentor Shaun worked the stripper cage?

You're entitled to that feeling, of course.

But here's the real shocker: I was only a few years removed from being too ashamed of my body to even leave my dorm room. Those insecurities are pretty close to the surface even today, and back then, they were even closer. Scratch my skin and I still feel that hurt.

So, it was a kind of validation to have somebody say that they will pay you to expose that skin, because it doesn't look half bad. When you think of it, I was already doing that in a Broadway-style musical about God's top-ten laws. It had to be acceptable, minus a few more inches of fabric, at an L.A. club.

No, you can't find clips of me at Crow Bar on YouTube. I hope.

But that job, at age 25, was another kind of a breakthrough moment.

You probably wouldn't blame me if I'd been a little confused about sex—gay, hetero, or otherwise—after the initiation I had at age 8. I might have hidden from sex entirely as an adult, or gotten trapped in a repeat cycle of abuse myself.

I didn't let either of those things happen to me. When I went on at the Crow Bar, I felt the power of the performer. I was in control of what I did, and audiences were reacting to *my* choices. It allowed me to reclaim sex for myself—as a man, as a dancer, as an individual who was free to chart his own course in bed, onstage, and in life.

And notice I didn't say "gay man."

When I married Scott a few years ago—thank you, U.S. Supreme Court—a small but noisy portion of my social media followers ripped me for it. That's predictable, but I was also a little shocked to see that people were disappointed by the realization that I was off the market by marriage *and* by sexual preference.

"What a waste of a man," they'd say, in disappointment, as if they had a shot at dating every man in the world, including me.

Oh, please.

With all the noise about gay marriage and sexual identity and coming out in recent years, I feel like people are making too much of a choice that is entirely private.

I'm not a gay workout teacher, and *INSANITY* won't help you get gay abs. As your trainer, I want you to do better and feel better about who you are.

"Sexy" has a million definitions, and every one of them is entirely personal. Which is the wonderful thing about it.

Being gay and being straight are equally mysterious and amazing ways to see the world, and they play out in private between two people who are maybe just in lust with each other. It's even better when they're in love.

But, for the majority of the time, most of us are just people, out of the sack and living our lives. We are so many things in addition to our sexual preferences. Saying that "gay" or "straight" defines you makes about as much sense as saying your hair color defines you.

And, that's a good thing, because sometimes I shave all of mine off.

When people rip me online for my sexuality, I just turn it back on them. One of my most popular Facebook posts ever came in response to a fan who just couldn't accept my marriage to Scott.

"Someone called me a 'fag' on social media," I wrote. "I don't really care what people think of me because *I am who I am*. Gay doesn't define me. I define me. If you don't like my positivity, encouragement, and belief, don't visit my pages, don't buy my programs, and don't hate on me. I'm not changing for you, I'm changing for the better. At least I'm trying."

A hundred thousand people hit the "like" or "love" button after I posted.

I hope the guy learned something from my response, plus the supportive notes from my followers on Facebook. Hate can be instructive when you're willing to examine it—it's like a roadblock on your personal GPS that you need to figure out. A lot of the time, it comes from a place that's so dark and so covered up that it makes people run screaming in the opposite direction. So, if a picture of Scott and me on Instagram makes you squirm, it's time to figure out why.

Calling somebody a "fag" might give you a little emotional release, but it won't help you understand why you need that release. The stronger your feelings are, the more important it is for you to deal with them.

I can let that word—*fag*—roll off me now. I don't even care. I feel sorry for the people who use it as a weapon, because it usually means that they're suffering from something that they can't face.

Earlier in my life, I tried hiding from myself, and I tried to meet the expectations of others, but I just couldn't. The only thing that did work was honesty. Being real. Learning from my discomfort and accepting myself.

Maybe you'll be lucky enough to have somebody throw a slur at you some day. I hope it reminds you that you need to define yourself before somebody else tries slap a label on you that doesn't fit.

I WAS BOOKED INTO A TOURING production of *Hello, Dolly!* but I never even made it to the first rehearsal. My greatest fear became a reality: Shaun T, the professional dancer, twisted his ankle stepping off a curb.

Hello, Dolly! went off to Indiana (or was it Tennessee?) without me, and I was 100 percent devastated. Plus, feeling vulnerable, because if my ankle didn't work, I didn't either. The orthopedist strapped my ankle into a walking boot, and I headed for the couch, flexing my hurt ankle and my fear of what I would do while I healed. Naturally, that's when my agent called, speaking words I never believed I'd hear: "Mariah Carey wants you to dance with her."

"When is the audition?"

Now I'm glaring at my hurt foot.

My agent said, "There's no audition. She picked you from your picture."

Which picture?

The one from the rooftop in New York.

Before any of this L.A. stuff happened to me.

Before I even knew I could make it as a dancer.

Before I had anything at all going for me, except a passion for dancing and a determination to prove my ex-boyfriend wrong.

TRUTHBOMB: You never know when a small gesture of belief in yourself might end up convincing the most important person in your world that you have what it takes.

Of course, Mariah Carey wasn't really *in* my world. The closest I had gotten to her up until that point was that her song woke me up every morning as a teenager. She recorded "Outside," and now she had invited me inside her troupe of dancers.

When I hung up the phone, it hit me. If I had traveled with the touring show of *Hello, Dolly!* I wouldn't have been available for the gig with Mariah.

But, when someone says I was lucky, I say, "You don't know how hard I worked to get to that moment!"

I don't deny some fortunate (ankle) twists and kind (abdominal) cuts, but I also insist that even those came from choices I made and work I did to put me in a position to be lucky.

It wasn't a bolt of lightning that struck the day Mariah Carey called. Instead, it was the culmination of working daily to overcome my obstacles, the skill I piled on skill, the hours I had spent doing every job that came my way and always looking for more, to the point where I could be sitting around with an ankle boot on and get a phone call from the most inspiring person in my life.

TRUTHBOMB: It isn't about the breakthrough. It's about doing the work that allows you to break *through*.

And, that's why I tell people in my classes: "In the 30 minutes that you work out, *go for it*." You won't ever hear me say, "Oh yeah, I'm going to do something leisurely."

No. I'm *eating*. Because that's the only attitude that has ever worked for me my entire life.

You know the expression "When one door closes, another opens"? Well, I stuck my sore ankle in a soundstage door, and Mariah Carey walked through it. Oh, I threw that walking boot off right quick in advance of that gig. Medical miracle.

The call for dancers was at 11:00 in the morning. We were supposed to work through the number before Mariah showed up, so we could be efficient with her time.

We ran through the dance a few times, burning off the nervous energy.

I was playing it cool and professional, but inside, I was so excited that I could barely stand it. My life goal realized!

I'm thinking: *Okay, at least she's gonna show up, and I'm gonna get over this nervousness, and then I'll be able to perform the rest of the day.*

Just, not quite yet.

We waited awhile. The clock ticked past noon. No Mariah.

We danced again, just to stay warm. No pulled muscles now, you hear?

The door didn't open.

Lunch break. Another warm-up, another wait.

Afternoon sun slanting through the studio windows. All quiet.

The sun set, dinnertime came and went, and the clock just kept on ticking.

Then, word from Mariah!

She'd been delayed.

No. Really?

So, we waited some more.

Eventually, 11:00 p.m. rolled around, and the studio door swung open. A small figure appeared in the doorway. I don't think she even said anything. She just opened her mouth and sang.

And that was enough for Shaun T.

I said to myself, "This is the voice of an angel."

As good as her recordings are? They don't do that voice justice.

To be in the room, and have Mariah's pure sound wash over me, I knew I had been accepted, finally.

It's not that she gave that gift to me. But rather, I knew I had earned acceptance from *myself.*

Fifteen minutes later, she was gone.

It was a day well spent.

I HAD A FEW GIGS WITH Mariah in 2005. We did the World Music Awards that year, and the MTV Music Awards. I danced with her in a Pepsi commercial. I don't drink it now, but Pepsi was the one for me back then.

If you find the videos on YouTube, you'll see me keeping my professional cool, staying in the moment. But, with my dance career at its most visible point, it was also coming to an end.

It's not like I set out planning to retire from dancing.

To this day, I feel like I left something out there on the dance floor. If Janet Jackson called me up tomorrow and wanted me to help her re-create her Velvet Rope tour, I'd be out the door before you could say, "Where's Shaun?"

But, while I was backing up Mariah, another career chose me. You know which one I'm talking about, because, if you're reading this book, you probably know me as a workout guy more than a dancer.

A trainer friend at Equinox—you see how this works yet?—called one day and said words that would change my life. Maybe yours, too.

"One of my clients works for Beachbody, and she wants to do a program with you. Can I give her your number?"

And, that's how I ended up talking to Lara Ross.

There was that time when Lewis met Clark. When Gladys Knight met the Pips. When Michelle met Barack. When M met M.

So it was when Shaun T met Lara and Beachbody, and 10,000 stronger cores were born. Or, more important, when a million people looked in the mirror and said, "Shaun's right: *I can do this.*"

In hindsight, I can connect the dots from today back into my past.

Each of us is our very own dot connector, when we look from now into the future. We can plot every point up to the current moment, but it's up to us to envision the line forward. Not only that, we need to ensure that there will be a next dot, rather than stopping before you make the most important connections and greatest leaps forward.

To avoid *that* fate, we need to develop the imagination to place another point out there, and build the strength to leap onto it. The gap may be scary, but the alternative is even scarier—that we'll be stuck in this place for the rest of our lives. Plenty of time for that at the cemetery.

So, I ask you: Where's you next landing place?

I'll meet you out there.

T IS FOR TRANSFORMATION

SUPERPOWER #4: FLEXIBILITY

Just as having a flexible body frees you up for yoga, being a flexible person frees you up to bend your life past the hard parts. Failure or f'ups won't throw you—at least not for long. You'll be able to develop a new strategy and move on. When Plan A doesn't work, you'll move on to Plan B, C, D, and E—or Z—when you need to.

SELF-TEST:
HOW FLEXIBLE ARE YOU?

[1 = That's me! 6 = That's totally not me!]

1. When I make a plan, I hang with it to the death.

1	2	3	4	5	6

2. Failure sticks with me like toilet paper on a boot heel.

1	2	3	4	5	6

3. When my mind is made up, it's my way or the highway.

1	2	3	4	5	6

4. I stick with my plan, even if it's not working.

1	2	3	4	5	6

5. I just want to be consistent.

1	2	3	4	5	6

SCORE BOX

Mostly 1s and 2s: Stiff!

Mostly 3s and 4s: You're hanging loose, but you could stand to be even looser.

Mostly 5s and 6s: Okay, you can bend, but can you hold solid when you need to?

SHAUN T'S
FLEX WORKOUT

EXERCISE #1

Stretch yourself. If you scan the back row in my *CIZE* workouts, you'll see one of my favorite dancers in the world. A guy named Pablo. A few years back, he weighed more than 300 pounds. Then his mom invited him to join her doing *Hip*

Hop Abs. Two years later, and 150 pounds lighter, he posted video to #shauntfitness, dancing like he was born in a chorus line. That's how I met him, and why I invited him to *CIZE* it up with me. New ideas can be like Pablo's mom: They help you break old habits and make you stretch for new ways of living that you never dreamed were possible. Just ask Pablo.

"Stretching" Exercises

Like, literally, stretch! You know I'm all about physical analogies to states of mind, and I truly believe that if your body becomes more flexible, your mind will match it. You free yourself in a whole new way the first time you drop down and touch your toes, or when you place two hands on your lower back and open your chest. A yoga class will help get you there. But, while you're shopping for tights and a yoga mat (and a teacher), try my two favorite stretches.

Child's pose: A yoga move where you drop to the floor, fold your knees under you, drop your torso onto your thighs, and extend your hands forward to press against the floor.

Rotational stretch: Bend slightly at the knees and waist, rotate one ankle up onto the opposite thigh, and then ease into a squat as you bring your palms together in front of your chest.

Scott does these two poses before bed every night to stretch his back and work out the kinks from his day of desk work and phone chatter.

EXERCISE #2

Stretch your mind. Meet people who are different than you are. If you're a high-school English teacher, sign up for the technical convention in the next city over. If you're an accountant, sign up for a watercolor class. If you're an athlete, join a book group. If you're a meat-and-potatoes person, find something to eat at the vegan restaurant. The surest way to introduce new ideas is to go to new places and meet the people who hang out there. If you invest the time to learn new perspectives, new ideas—and creative connections between them—will follow.

EXERCISE #3

Goof off. A lot of us berate ourselves for flipping around the TV dial or browsing through web sites and magazines. First of all, do it because your brain needs a break from all that intense concentration. But, also do it because picking up a bit of this and a snatch of that can open your mind to new pathways, and that's where the creative ideas are. Steve Jobs often credited a calligraphy course he took for the ideas that led to the development of the iPhone. He's calling *you*.

EXERCISE #4

Get back out there. I see a lot of people plodding through a lot of routine workouts and not getting anywhere. But, when there's a game on the line, they push themselves just a little bit farther in the spirit of competition. Remember that game you killed at in high school, but gave up, even though you loved it? Sign up for a team, and push yourself again. Not up to full-court in basketball yet? How about beach volleyball or even bowling? Or, you could *CIZE* it up with Pablo and me. Again, you'll need to work within your capabilities at present. But there are beginners' classes everywhere, and once you start, you'll stretch beyond your comfort zone.

EXERCISE #5

Go back to school. One of the most immediate places you can stretch is between your ears. Your brain is infinitely expandable. The more you cram into it the bigger it gets. Take a language, or learn how to play an instrument. Brain studies show that people who push themselves mentally in middle age stay sharp as oldsters.

EXERCISE #6

Build your empathy. What does this have to do with flexibility? Everything. The more you see and understand other people's problems—mentoring a high-school kid, or delivering food to people who need it, like my Pop-Pop and I did—the more you stretch beyond your own prejudices and preconceived notions. Sticking in your little circle shrinks your world. Volunteering stretches you beyond it.

EXERCISE #7

Forgive yourself. People who are inflexible to the outside world are often tough on themselves, inside. The best way to tell is if you are constantly talking yourself down over your failures and screw-ups. Then you need language lessons in better self-talk. Think of it this way: You should be speaking to yourself the same way you would if you were consoling or counseling a close friend. Be there for *you* first. And, the more support you give yourself, the more likely you are to expand your world and engage with others.

EXERCISE #8

Get lost on purpose. You've heard that travel broadens your life, your knowledge, your interests. But, that doesn't mean you have to take a cruise to Helsinki. You can "travel" if you simply make time to listen to a podcast host you know you disagree with, order takeout from a restaurant you've never tried before, or book an Airbnb in a nearby neighborhood you've never visited. Being open to new experiences is a key flexibility builder, and the more of them you have, the flexier you'll be.

And, If You're Too Flexible

For those of you who logged too many 5s and 6s above, here's how to develop a backbone, in three easy lessons.

1. **Take your time over decisions.** The more you think about your decisions, the more likely you'll develop a position you'll stick to.

2. **Practice saying "no."** Using that word is an opportunity to reclaim your life. Use it politely, but often. The boundaries you build expand your own opportunities.

3. **Put yourself on a schedule.** I mean, literally, put the things *you* need, *you* desire, *you're* curious about, on your daily schedule—three workouts a week, time to read before bed, a getaway with friends at the end of the summer. If you don't schedule the important things in your life, other people will fill that time for you. Don't let them!

CHAPTER THIRTEEN

BEFORE THE "BEFORE," AND AFTER THE "AFTER"

People in the fitness industry seem to love "before and after" pictures. I even see them in my own infomercials, and they always make me wonder.

TRUTHBOMB: It's more important what comes before the "before" picture and what comes after the "after" picture.

If you're living your "before" picture right now, I'll hug you just the same as I would if you're the best "after" you'll ever be. Both of those folks may need a lot of love, especially from themselves.

Before the "before," maybe you're living with a past you haven't been able to face or delivering self-talk that lays you flat all day long. Or maybe you're still hurting from unspeakable loss that you have to compensate for somehow.

No matter how big you were before you started working out, or how tiny you were after you completed a program, it's the person you are now that I care about. It's the person you were before you resolved to make a change who is the most important, because that is the person living the pain, the doubt, and the helplessness that you're going to have to work through.

Your before the "before" person deserves the utmost respect, too, because that is who will launch you on the journey to who you want to become. When you snap that "before" picture, it is because your "before" self mustered the strength to commit to a new phase of the journey.

That's a show of strength like no other.

So, the "after" photo is better, right? Showing off the "new" you and all that?

I don't want to scare anybody, but after the "after" is where the real work begins. As difficult as it can be to lose weight, it's even harder to lock in a new lifestyle that satisfies you for the rest of your life. If you haven't done the necessary work to transform yourself inside, it will begin to show up again on the outside, and yo-yo weight loss and gain, or other retreats into bad habits, can be devastating.

Shaun T has troubles with his "after" too, in case you were wondering. Some days, I'm searching for that will to continue as much as you are.

Y'all need to know Darren Natoni. He's one of my circle-of-five guys, and he travels with me on *Shaun T Live* events, in part because you can't slow the guy down or shut him up. He's relentlessly positive and upbeat.

It's exhausting to have him as a workout partner, of course.

Recently, we were in about day 43 of *INSANITY*—far from the end, deep in exhaustion—and about to do a workout. I was in a lousy mood and heading for the bathroom. It wasn't because I had to go particularly. More like I wanted to hide from Darren.

He wouldn't have any part of that attitude, and called me on it. "You need to change your mindset," he told me. "Instead of saying, 'This is gonna be really hard,' you need to say, 'I'm going to attack this. I'm going to look at this as a challenge. I'm gonna kick its butt before it ever has a chance to kick mine.'"

Leave me alone, Darren!

I especially hate it when he says stuff like that, because he's right!

So, I turned back to the work and my discomfort zone. It's the only place I've ever accomplished anything worth doing. (And, by the way, if you want Darren to hassle you, I'd be happy to pass him on. Anything to get him off my case!)

I'm not just talking about physical strength here, of course. The specific movement doesn't matter. It could be a half-tuck jump you execute in minute 23 of *FOCUS T25*, or it could be an accounting course you take in night school. Either way, you're adding strength, which makes you feel better *and* prepares you to grow even stronger. It's your force multiplier, your stairway to awesome.

The key question is: Do you have the tools you need to be happy and sustain that happiness? If not, you'll have to find, and finally deal with, the reasons that caused you to gain weight, or lose the job, or fail in the relationship, in the first place.

True transformation starts before the "before" and continues long after the "after."

TRUTHBOMB: No photograph can capture the most important work, because it happens *inside*.

IN MY WORKOUTS, THE MODIFIER SHOWS a lower-impact version of the workout. The misconception is that it's who you follow if you're weak, if you're a beginner, if you're barely after the "before" photo.

Right?

The whole idea is to be strong, to kick ass, to kick your own ass, if necessary. Right?

Wrong, wronger, and wrongest. Listen up: I *began* my career as a DVD fitness coach as a modifier!

You heard that right.

I was introduced something like this: "And now, meet your fitness motivator and exercise modifier . . . *Charles T!*"

Wait. Who?

That's me on my first fitness DVD *All the Right Moves,* appearing as the not-so-famous Charles T.

The lead trainer was Grace Lazenby, and I was the dude in the back right, sitting in a chair, demonstrating moves for people who needed a low-impact alternative to the full workout.

Why the name change?

Grace's buddy, another guy named Shaun—he even spelled it like my name—was in the front row, and she wasn't going to make *him* change it up for the video. So, I went by my middle name, given in honor of my Pop-Pop. And, I was damn excited about working with Grace and other-Shaun, too. Call me anything. Just let me show up on a fitness DVD!

Grace kept calling out: "Those of you who need to take it a little easier, watch Charles, in the chair. . . ."

Cut to me, super-serious, doing my body-saving best.

I love that guy Charles, sitting in the chair. He had no idea what was going to come next. He was just grateful to Grace for another step along the road, and you have to love all of those next steps, wherever they may lead.

It's perfect that I'm the modifier on that workout, of course.

Think of it, I've cast Tania as a modifier, and she was one of my first pals in the business of dance and exercise. Scott was the modifier on *INSANITY Max 30*, along with Danielle Natoni, who people call the female Shaun T. These are the most capable people I know, so I entrust them with the most important audience for a Shaun T workout: The people who may need a slightly different path.

TRUTHBOMB: If you're new to a workout, or a life phase, you are working harder, suffering more, and earning the biggest gains. The new people are by far the strongest people who are doing my workouts, because they're closest to "before."

Modifier pride! I love you guys! Go, Charles T, go!

He really wasn't ready to be the headliner just yet.

When my buddy at Equinox hooked me up with Lara Ross, I walked into it with my eyes wide open and my brain mostly empty. It was just another new thing in the midst of a million other new things I was trying out in L.A., so I'd figure it out as I went along.

Lara wanted me to do a screen test, teaching a class. So I cleared out the garage in the house I was sharing at that time, and moved every mirror I could find down there, where the lawnmower used to be. I invited some friends over (including Tania), and we went for it, developing the workout that would become *Hip Hop Abs*. Before I encouraged America to tilt, tuck, and tighten—my signature phrase back then—a group of friends did it with me in a garage in Sherman Oaks.

Putting together this workout was an amazing opportunity, and it was also something I'd been doing several times a day, every day, since my sophomore year at Rowan. So, my big opportunity came back then, not when Lara Ross invited me to be filmed by Beachbody.

Lara watched my tape, then told me they'd like to work with me to develop a DVD for Beachbody. She sent over a contract, and I passed it on to the agent who was handling my dance gigs.

There was just one thing he took exception to. My contract stipulated that I'd get a certain percentage of sales if I appeared in an infomercial, but according to my agent, it was already doomed. "Infomercials never work," he told me. "We don't want to tie our income to that money, because there won't be any."

Basically, my agent opted out of his share in any earnings from my infomercials going forward.

I shrugged—well, *okay*—and left the office. By the time I reached the parking lot, I was pissed. "You don't trust and believe in me," I thought, "when I've shown you that I'm really good?"

I wasn't in this for infomercial money or DVD sales or to become a famous trainer on TV. I was doing it for the same reason that drove me the first time I'd stepped in front of a fitness class: **If I can help just one person, it will be worth it.**

That's true to this day, whether I'm working out with 15 people, or 15,000. And, I remain grateful to that agent, and not just because the infomercial income turned out to be substantial after all. Money isn't everything, but it *is* something, right?

But because, in a sense, the agent did me a solid by telling me that my new initiative with Beachbody was going to fail. It took away all of the pressure.

It wasn't going to be a success, anyway, right? So, I wasn't going to change anything about the way I approached the new gig. To me, teaching was about motivating through movement, and reaching the person who was doing the movement. What kept them in the moment? What made them push a little harder than they did yesterday? That was my whole agenda, and I wasn't changing it up for Beachbody or *any*body.

We went into the brainstorming process for the new workout, and *Hip Hop Abs* was born. Another tip of the operating-room cap to my abdominal surgeon, who operated on my burst appendix and avoided giving me a big old zipper from navel to sternum. Couldn't have done it without you, man.

I wasn't intimidated by the production process. I would simply develop my program, then teach a class—things I'd done a thousand times before—projecting toward the video cameras while I did it. The lenses were my audience, so I might as well have been at the nuclear power plant in Jersey. The goal was the same: teaching engineers and secretaries how to dance. I just couldn't see them yet.

After a whirlwind experience shooting, I went back to my regular life. I wasn't holding my breath for my video to take off. My agent had made sure to set my expectations nice and low. I just went about my business. If your only goals are to help one person at a time and push yourself along the way, you don't need a lot of gear to achieve it.

One Saturday, Lara Ross called me to say, "We're testing the infomercial today."

I didn't feel any anxiety. I was just excited. Something new!

The next morning, she called up and said, "Your financial problems are over." A lot of people wanted to have *Hip Hop Abs*, evidently. The orders were clicking in.

I was happy, of course, but I wasn't thinking about those dollars flowing into my checking account. I was simply excited that now I could connect to more people who had been where I'd been and needed a lift.

I knew what it was like to be overweight.

I knew what it was like to be insecure.

I knew what it was like to not fit into a pair of jeans that I fit into last week.

I knew what it was like to step onto the scale and fear what it would tell me.

I knew what it felt like to not want to take my shirt off at the beach.

I also knew what it took to get past all of that, so I could motivate others to do the same. And, then, we could celebrate together.

I'd been before the "before," and I was living after the "after." I still think it's the reason why I've been able to make a career out of transformations—first my own, and then yours.

My real reward for *Hip Hop Abs* came about 8 weeks after the launch of the DVD. I typed in the URL for an infomercial-review web site, and searched for *Hip Hop Abs*. Boom! People were seeing results, talking about how confident they were becoming, talking about how much fun they were having.

I had reached my one person, times several thousand, and those were the numbers that really counted. I've lived on food stamps, I've lived paycheck to paycheck, and I've had enough money to appreciate the truth behind Notorious B.I.G.'s "Mo Money, Mo Problems."

Cash can buy me something to eat or take me on a vacation or buy me a house to live in. But, all these things can be burned down or stolen, or the vacation ends after 2 weeks and I'm miserable because I don't wanna leave. Money is just a transaction, no different from swiping your card for a coffee at Dunkin' Donuts. Drink that coffee, and it's *over*.

I can tell you for sure that the only real gold is what you hold inside of you—the lessons you've learned, the achievements you've celebrated, and the people you celebrate with, because nobody can take those away from you.

The more you connect with people, the more everything else falls into place. Financially it will work, emotionally it will work, and you'll free your mind of negativity, because positive things are happening.

Here's one that I keep in my Shaun T safe deposit box:

Beachbody sent me into a QVC studio in Canada to talk to people about *Hip Hop Abs*. A funny lady came on the input line, all full of laughter and appreciation for the program.

"I've lost 35 pounds working out with you, Shaun. You crack me up!"

She was cracking me up, too, and I told her so.

Then, she said, "I'm going to keep on losing weight *in my wheelchair*. When you pump to the right, I roll to the right. And, when you pump left, I roll to the left. Thank you, Shaun T!"

Who was thanking who?

To me, that exchange is all the payback I ever need from my life in fitness.

And, in fact, there was another ripple of satisfaction underneath the success of *Hip Hop Abs* as well. I hadn't tried anything crazy with it. I hadn't worked outside what I knew. I just brought it to a new place. If you can succeed that way, without leaving the real you behind, you're wealthy indeed.

BUT I DID BUY ONE NEW TOY.

Focusina had been acting up. I felt like that movie cowboy who rides his old horse all the way out West, and then releases her into the clover field. But, I'd looked into that broken rearview mirror one time too many. I'd always dreamed of owning a Ford F-150 truck, so I drove Focusina to Sunrise Ford of North Hollywood on Lankershim Boulevard. I said goodbye to Focusina, and drove off in a truck with a much better rearview mirror.

My future was coming on strong and fast at that point in 2007.

With *Hip Hop Abs* rocking the infomercial world, it wasn't long before Beachbody came back to me for another dance-themed workout: *Rockin' Body*. And, as a kid who'd been through a bumpy patch of childhood, nobody had to ask me twice to produce *Get Real with Shaun T*, which focused on diabetes prevention for teenagers, and *Shaun T Fit Club*, for the under-10 set.

Then, in June 2008, Beachbody CEO Carl Daikeler was looking for a trainer to lead a program called *INSANITY*. My favorite adjective is "crazy," so I thought I might be a fit.

I threw my hat in the ring, and Carl tossed it back out. "You're our dance guy, Shaun. This is for *athletes*."

Quiz: What's the one thing you can say to Shaun T to give him extra motivation?

I wouldn't accept Carl's decision, so I met with him in a conference room at Beachbody's offices in Santa Monica. I asked, "What do you want this *INSANITY* thing to be?"

He fired back, "What do *you* think it should be? Show me what you got."

I was like, "Did you just challenge me?"

Motivation, round two.

The next morning, I woke up at 5:00 and wrote up the very first version of Cardio Power and Resistance, which are the keys to the *INSANITY* workout. I asked myself, "What did I feel like on my first day of track-and-field in high school?" That was when I discovered what peak physical conditioning feels like, and it changed me forever.

Back in Chapter Four, I told you how Coach Anderson kicked my ass, and transformed it, on the first day of track practice. Everything we did that day found its way into *INSANITY*. He ran me through hell for 30 days—you might even say it was *insane*—but, by the time we were 60 days out, I started winning races.

That exact progression—from "I can't possibly" . . .

. . . to "Oh my God, this hurts,"

. . . to "I'm going to show that guy,"

. . . to "Hey, I'm getting stronger,"

. . . to "This is the best I've felt in my whole life!"

. . . is exactly what I wanted *INSANITY* to be.

So, I built the workout on paper, I invited a test group of

my fittest friends to meet me at a dance studio, and turned on the camera.

They all thought they were going to dance.

Welcome to Coach Sonny Anderson track practice, yo!

I started jogging, and there were nervous glances around the room. But, when I introduced the diamond jumps and switch kicks, there were gasps and complaints. I kept moving forward. At the end of 30 minutes, I was the only one standing.

To the extent that they could still talk, my friends wheezed out, "You are *ridiculous*. That was *crazy*."

Exactly.

But was it *INSANITY*?

I dropped the DVD off with Carl.

"Here's the workout," I told him, and left.

No sales job from me. Either he wanted a workout that would push people to the limit, or he didn't.

The next day, his response was equally simple, "This program is *yours*."

Credit where it's due: Carl not only motivated me, he was willing to look at me in a new way and give me a new opportunity. His "dance guy" was about to move to a whole new level of training, but he was flexible enough to see that I had a lot to offer outside of the category he knew me for. And that title—*INSANITY*—was magic. In fact, a lot of the exercise videos that were out at that time were all about "easy" and "in just 2 weeks."

This one would change the face—and body—of fitness.

People were about to meet a whole new me. The party boy of *Hip Hop Abs* was replaced by Shaun T-is-for-tough-trainer. But the new workout matched where I was in my life. It had to, for it to work the way I wanted it to.

I looked deeper into myself, and asked, "How did I get through my life? How did I push past hard times?"

The first and most obvious answer came in my early years of track-and-field, when I was about to throw up during a workout. *INSANITY* had to be crazy hard, because that was the name. Obviously.

But, it went deeper. I wanted it to challenge people so they'd need to call on inner motivation. It wasn't about being swept along by the music, like with *Hip Hop Abs*. Now, people would be hurting and tempted to quit every step of the way.

I'd been there, too, at so many times in my life. I could have said, "I can't deal" and walked off the field or back into the bedroom. Or, I could find another level of effort and push back. That was the essential exercise I wanted people to master with *INSANITY*: Pushing back against the temptation to quit.

Around this time, I moved from L.A. to New York. It was kind of an *INSANITY*-driven move, in fact. All of the test groups for my other workout programs had been in L.A., and they had gone fine. But, I was trying to tap into another vibe now, something grittier, more real, closer to the bone. True for the workout, true for me as well. I gave up the 405 Freeway and opted for the subway instead. Less sunshine, more city. Less laid back, more life on the run. I was back on the track, after 5 years in a traffic jam.

For me as a sprinter, there was no equipment out there. I didn't have a ball to throw through a hoop or a helmet and pads to crash into people with. It was just me in a flimsy track uniform, trying to throw my body forward.

To this day, during a workout, I'm always all about: Can we please get to the point where I can't breathe? The rest just seems like a waste of time. That's why I push you: I don't want either of us to waste your precious time.

It makes me think of track practice in another way as well.

INSANITY is the ultimate challenge. It steals your breath fast, because it's based entirely on body-weight exercises. It's just you, feeling the pain, but lifting yourself up. It forces you to say, "This is my body. It's all I have. And, I'm going to push it until it breaks, or gets stronger."

So, there's Shaun leaning into the camera, or crouching down during a *Shaun T Live* event, looking you right in the eye, and dropping a . . .

TRUTHBOMB: If you can hold up your body, you can hold up your life.

So difficult. But that's what makes it so powerful.

And, as you hold up your body, and your life, you appreciate something I learned on the track practice field:

TRUTHBOMB: There is always, *always* a reserve. If your body says "quit," but your mind says "I . . . CAN . . . DO . . . THIS," you're laying down the strength that will serve you for a lifetime.

The only way to get through *INSANITY* is to constantly pass that relay baton over the course of 60 days. (Well, actually *63* days, which is my little *INSANITY* joke on everybody who does the program. What, you don't find that funny?) Every X through a calendar day is a new challenge met, and each day when you wake up, there's another challenge to tackle.

Will you earn another X, or give in? Will you pass the baton, or drop it?

When you place that final X on the last calendar page, it's the ultimate feeling. Sure, you'll feel stronger than you ever have in your life. But more important, you will have triumphed over the urge to quit.

And, that's superpower you can apply to any challenge.

DURING A BREAK FROM SHOOTING THE *INSANITY* DVD, I took a vacation to Majorca, Spain.

I had been with Mom-Mom just a few weeks before, and I noticed that, when we were out together, she needed to take a breather when normally she'd be striding out ahead of everybody. But she was still Mom-Mom. Maybe I thought somebody who was *that* strong could never die. We had something special going, especially since that first night I spent at their house, at age 14. After Pop-Pop died, when I was in my early twenties, I was in charge of helping Mom-Mom enjoy life a little more.

I taught her how to swear—sometimes even the minister's wife just gotta say "damn!"—and I took her out shopping to buy her first pair of slacks: hunter-green sweats. (Back in the day, proper ministers' wives wore skirts and dresses only.) It was cool to see her actually feel comfortable for a change.

"Shauny, you're a terrible influence on me!" she told me back then. But, she didn't mean it. Probably. Nobody else could get her to relax! I owed her so much. She taught me how to scramble eggs! She made me Campbell's tomato soup after school, and dropped an ice cube in so it wouldn't burn my mouth.

And, she made me feel safe at home for the first time in my life, at age 14.

Now, our relationship was in its final days.

My mom tracked me down in Spain. I could tell something was wrong from the sound of her voice. "If you want to see Mom-Mom again, you better come home." I went straight to the airport, and then to Mom-Mom's home. There, I found Ennis washing her arms and forehead. He was a saint to her at the end.

I was devastated to see how far she had fallen since my last visit. I put my hand on her arm and said, "Mom-Mom, can you please just open your eyes? I need to see you one more time."

Ennis said, "Mom-Mom, Shaun is here."

And then, a miracle happened.

Her eyes flickered open, and she gave a small smile and wave.

It was the last time she opened her eyes.

I stayed in the house for the next couple of days, sleeping on the floor by her bed. I played Mom-Mom's favorite gospel songs and sang along. She was breathing gently and seemed at peace.

Eventually I had to leave the house. I had to film the second part of *INSANITY*, and the crew and exercisers were waiting for me. But I was strong enough to go on, because the lady who had taught me the real meaning of strength had looked into my eyes one last time.

She died 2 days later.

And she's still with me every day.

When there are people and experiences that give you strength, you need to install them as permanent co-pilots in the front seat with you.

It's kind of like the St. Christopher statues people mount on their dashboards. In my mind, I have a miniature Mom-Mom up there as well, pointing the way forward.

T IS FOR TRANSFORMATION

SUPERPOWER #5: SELFISHNESS

You've completed a lot of exercises now, and I hope it's helping you develop an agenda for what you want to accomplish. I guarantee you that the more ambitious your goals, the more obstacles there will be to achieving them. The most difficult obstacles will be human ones. That's right, all the people who are satisfied to have you in just the position you are and don't want you to change a thing, because it will be inconvenient for them if you do!

This is where a little selfishness will come in handy.

I didn't take a vote among my friends whether I should move to L.A. I did it because it was right for me. I was selfish with my goals, and that led to some game-changers in my life. Every day begins and ends with you. So, be a little selfish. Instead of blaming other people for what's happening to you, or waiting for them to push you forward, ask yourself: What did I do for *myself* today to change the game?

SELF-TEST:
ARE YOU SELFISH ENOUGH?

Rate yourself for each of the statements below.

[1 = That's me! 6 = That's totally not me!]

1. I'm an unpaid chauffeur for everyone I know.

1	2	3	4	5	6

2. If I miss my kids' school events or games, I feel guilty!

1	2	3	4	5	6

3. I get 3 weeks of vacation time at work, but I don't always take it.

1	2	3	4	5	6

4. At my office, I take orders instead of giving them.

1	2	3	4	5	6

5. My favorite stuff never makes it to the top of the to-do list.

1	2	3	4	5	6

SCORE BOX:

Mostly 1s and 2s: You're living for everybody *but* yourself.

Mostly 3s and 4s: You can be selfish, when others get out of the way.

Mostly 5s and 6s: Selfish to a fault. (But, is it a fault?)

SHAUN T'S
ALL-ABOUT-U! WORKOUT

EXERCISE #1: Take the inventory

- **Divide up the clock.** Very often, we let the schedule tell us what to do, rather than setting a schedule that meets our own needs. Keep a small notebook handy as you work through your days, and make a note of it every time you change activities. Add up where all those hours go. Then, you can take steps to budget those precious minutes better.

- **Determine who (and what) is wasting your time.** Use the same activity list, but mark it up with the primary people you do things for, if it's not you. Identifying time thieves is step one to reclaiming the precious thing that they take from you. Say: "Honey, would you please vacuum the basement?" "Kayley, after you do your homework, I need you to empty, then fill and run, the dishwasher." "Jackson, run down to the store and buy what's on the grocery list, will you? There's cash in my wallet." You *can* say these words, you know.

- **Decide what you want.** Pull out a sheet of paper, and list life goals that are exclusively yours. So, it's not "make sure that Kayley gets admitted to Princeton," but rather, "make sure I get my MBA before the next reorganization at work." (Less pressure: Learn to cook Italian, because dammit, that would be fun!) You don't have to be on track for the Nobel Peace Prize to have goals worth striving for. If they're *your* goals, carve out time for them! Write out four or five of them that a) are limited enough in scope that you can accomplish them in a year or so, and b) are realistic for you to fit into the schedule above. Now, plan your work, and work your plan.

EXERCISE #2: Learn the time-bandits' strategies (and counterattack them)

- **Keep your cool.** If people try to *bully* you into doing their work or running their errands, don't commit to anything, even if it's the fastest way to defuse a tense situation. Instead, take any time you need to collect yourself so that you can state your case for why you couldn't possibly do what they ask. Remember, these are thieves, so get 'em off your property. If you stick to your guns, they'll either do the job themselves (not likely) or find another victim (probably), but at least it won't be you.

- **Don't get sucked in.** If they try to *guilt* you into something that you'd rather not do, don't agree. Even if you've offered the kind of help that they're asking for in the past, calmly tell them that it's just not possible for you to help in that way anymore. You have responsibilities to yourself, and you need to get to them. Suggest an alternate strategy that could work for them, perhaps, then exit guilt-free.

- **Say no to whining.** If your time-waster tries to *pester* you into submission, tell him that you don't speak "whine" language, and that you won't do anything if they use that tone of voice. Leave the room if you have to. When the whining fails to get results, it'll stop, and their training for greater independence begins. Then, turn the task back on them; they'll figure it out, or they'll do without.

- **Know your priorities.** Perhaps the most insidious of all are people who try to *praise* you into doing their dirty work for them. It's called a feedback sandwich, where two compliments are wrapped around a stinky time suck that you're being asked to swallow. (Note the two slices of compliment around this request: "Gee, Claire, your property always looks so nice. Would you help me in my yard this weekend? Your trees are always pruned perfectly.") Thank them for the compliment, maybe even offer some advice on how you are able to keep the yard in such great shape, but then decline the heck out of that invitation. You have your own priorities; let them know that.

EXERCISE #3: Make plans, announce them, and stick to them

I would have to turn in my tough-trainer badge if I didn't say to start with your workouts! When you get busy, what's the first item of personal business that falls off the schedule? Your workout! The ultimate "you" time, when you take a walk, press play on a DVD workout, or head off to the gym. Don't let it happen to you! The best way to do that is to pull out the family calendar right now, and ink the workout time into place. Make sure that everybody knows that whatever is happening, it happens around that. You owe it to yourself, and you owe it to everybody in your life, that you maintain and improve your physical condition. Set that priority for yourself, explain it to others, and work the schedule so that they get the same privileges. Suddenly, you're all better off.

The same goes for your other priorities in your schedule. If your family knows that you have class every Wednesday night at 7:00, they'll find a way to do without you for those 2 hours. If you announce in April that you're going on a buddy trip or girlfriend getaway the third weekend in September, you're on record and the time becomes yours. (Make it an annual thing, and you're free that weekend for the *rest of your life!*) If Mommy and Daddy sit down for a glass of wine, alone, in a designated kid-free zone, every evening after work, the household will schedule itself around that tradition. And for goodness sake: Shut off the smartphone at night. When was the last time you received a truly urgent e-mail?

It's so important to make those kinds of commitments to yourself. Clearly block off the time that you need, and make sure that anybody who could interrupt you with their own needs is aware that you're off-limits for that period of time. It may take a little getting used to, but you will be so much better in the rest of your life when you designate a little bit of it just for yourself.

Are You Being Too Selfish?

Think about the difference between being selfish in the best way, and being a user in the worst way. Signs that selfishness has crossed the line:

- A user takes advantage of power discrepancies (parent over child, boss over subordinate, bully over pipsqueak) to force people to do stuff against their will. There is a difference between making everyone do their own work, delegating when you need help, and forcing others to do your work for you because you're in a position of power.

- A user manipulates the emotions (guilt, fear, shame) of her victim to ensure outcomes.

- A user doesn't look at the big picture, acting only in their own best interest and not considering how those actions will impact others.

- A user doesn't function as part of a team, tends not to collaborate with openness for everyone's ideas, never rolls up their sleeves and pitches in to benefit the greater good.

Do any of these apply to you? Ask the key people in your life for feedback, and don't plug your ears when they give it to you.

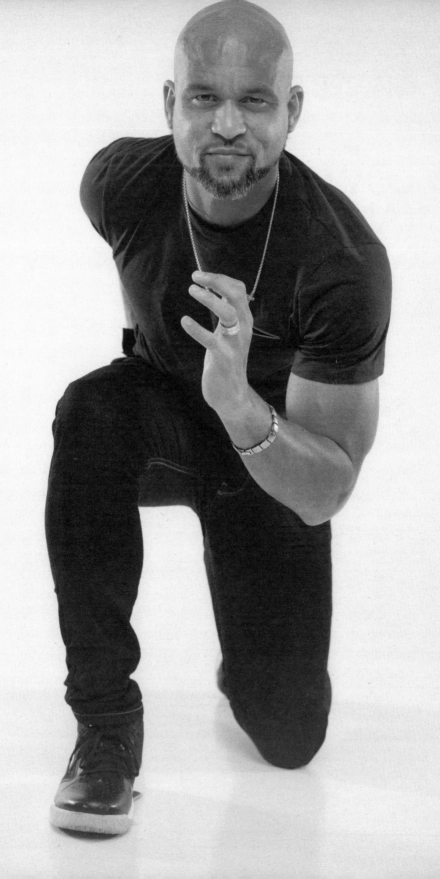

CHAPTER FOURTEEN

LOVING (AND HATING) *SHAUN T LIVE*

Sometimes, transformation is a group activity. That's why a lot of people like to exercise together, rather than on their own. You're strong for yourself, you're strong for others, and you can draw support from the group when you need it.

But a decline and fall can happen in a group, too. Human beings are social animals. We crave being with each other, for good and bad reasons. A group can become a mob if enough negative thinking takes over.

You probably know the bad side. You've seen haters attack somebody vulnerable online, and it's just like the playground in elementary school, except the bullies are hiding behind the anonymity of the Internet. But it happens in real life, too. Low-down people pull others down, because it gives them company in the muck.

The opposite is true, too, of course. Which is why I surround myself with people who lift me up—like Tania, Scott, Darren, Danielle, Jessica, Todd, and awesome Alex—when I'm doing my workouts. (You can never have too many amazing people in your circle of five!) They show me the best I can be, and remind me how I need to live, too.

That's why your Core Five are *so important* for you. They help you set the tone for everything you do, and it'll be a high tone, or a low one, depending on what music you're listening to.

Pump it up, okay?

I'M IN INDIANAPOLIS, THE DAY BEFORE Valentine's Day.

Another stop on the *Shaun T Live* tour. People who have done my workouts crave the chance to be together, suffer together, succeed together, and I want to be with them, too.

It's like extending my circle of 5 to a circle of 1,000, and the vibe is sky high.

An hour before the 9:00 a.m. kick-off, a line snakes through the lobby outside the venue, with people signing in for the event. They've come in packs of 3 or 10 or 15 to share the heat. Husbands and wives and boyfriends and girlfriends (or boyfriends, as the case may be) are out in support of each other. Some people are there alone.

There are a father and son, supporting each other in the battle against time.

I spot an alpha mom, topping off her alpha baby with alpha breast milk. It's so beautiful, I'm thinking: Maybe Shaun could work that out somehow, when Scott and I have children. (More about that next chapter.)

There are lots of girlfriend groups. At the Indy event, five ladies showed up in matching pink tank tops that said "Shaun T Is My Trainer. Who's Training YOU?" I asked them to send me one. I'm training them, they're motivating me. We all win.

I love everybody who shows up at my workouts. But, I throw an extra hug out to the people who show up and don't care if they look the part, or haven't lost the 40 pounds yet, or can't even hear what I'm saying from the stage.

I'm not making that last part up.

At an event in Jacksonville, I noticed a guy who was struggling through the workout. When I reached him and offered to help, he gestured to let me know he couldn't hear me. He was struggling but he wasn't leaving—he was still there doing the best that he could, given his hearing impairment. He stepped outside his comfort zone and communicated.

How amazing is that?

I got down on one knee and coached him for a little while, and he read my lips. We both lit up with that.

I ask again: Who's motivating who?

Think how brave you need to be to bring your imperfect self out in public and show a commitment that may only be *inside you* so far. A belief not yet a reality. Something you feel, but people can't see. Maybe you can't hang with all the steps. Maybe holding that plank is just a hope, not a possibility just yet. And yet you stand up in this group, and say: "I'm one of you. I belong here."

I embrace them. Everybody in my workouts does. Because we all started somewhere, and we all have somewhere to go.

IN A DIMLY LIT HALLWAY, BEFORE the Indy workout, I queue up my workout music, run some sprints to warm up, rock out to the music a little, and circle-hug with my team—Alex, Darren, Danielle, and my modifier-in-chief, Scott. In the huddle, I remind us that every person in the room needs support to trust and believe in who they are.

That's the real reason that we're gathered here: To share the journey, and to move it down the road another few steps.

I'm not nervous; I'm amped up. People are transforming their lives before my eyes, so the view is spectacular. I feel like I'm bursting out of the starting blocks at a relay, looking to put my teammates in the best possible position to grab the baton.

"How are you feeling, Indianapolis?"

From the sound of it, they're pretty hyped for 9:00 on a cold February morning in the Hoosier state.

First thing I do is read the energy in the room. What I really want to know is:

What's in their eyes.

How they lift their heads and try to focus.

Is someone scratching their head, tying their shoe?

Or, are they ready to sweat with me, and dig deeper with me?

When I shout, do they shout louder?

Are they nodding their heads, paying attention, snapping alive?

Most of the time, they're *crazy* with energy. People aren't here to march in place. They want to step it up to the next level.

Me, too.

Of course, some of the folks in Indy are a little nervous, hoping I'll take it easy on them.

Not me. Not now. It's time to get to work.

I can feel everybody revving up for the physical challenge, getting their blood moving, working their mojo. I am, too. We're all feeling what I remember from my prerace hype from track. Lots of muscle warmups, some random sprints in place, plus dozens of "insaniacs"—all different shapes and sizes—battening the hatches before the sweat hurricane.

We're all in for something difficult, and sharing it is just the point. We'll bond through boot camp.

One woman is wearing a tank top that reads: "I am fearfully and wonderfully made."

Which is crazy, because my grandfather loved to quote Psalm 139 to me. We hear you, Pop-Pop!

Another woman is wearing a T-shirt that proclaims: "I'm stronger than you think."

She believes in herself. And, that's the ultimate superpower, because she's lifting herself up and others, too, by example.

Recruit that spirit into your group. The best way to do that is to wear the shirt, and believe it yourself.

You *are* stronger than people think you are.

I know how lousy it feels to see a scary image in the mirror. And, I'm not done with that out-of-control feeling yet, not by a long shot. I still have a weakness for Dunkin' Donuts (the toasted coconut kind).

Been there. Now what?

These workouts are as much about tough questions as they are about physical challenges.

I'm calling out exercises of the mental *and* bodily kind.

Why do you want to lose weight?

What's holding you back?

Who's holding you back?

Can you love yourself more?

Can you accept who you are *right now*?

And, can you stick with this workout for a few more seconds today than you did yesterday?

We're in this as much for our hearts as we are for our bodies. I know this because of the questions I get during Q&A sessions.

It's not: Shaun, what's the proper form for a reverse lunge?

It's: What's the most difficult thing you've ever overcome?

Or: When I'm struggling with motivation, how can I keep going?

Or: How can I keep the haters and negative influences from dragging me down?

I wrestle with those questions every day.

During x-jumps, I remind everyone: "You gotta go down to go up."

The struggle to stay fit and the battle to lose weight are just two small parts of a bigger challenge: How do we stay true to ourselves in a world that can pull us down from every angle? We're all fighting gravity in this hotel ballroom, but we're also fighting it in our lives, to keep rising up. Muscle helps with that fight, but it's ultimately our minds that lift us up and keep us there.

Before the workout starts, my first instruction to the group is: "Hug someone you don't know." I pick out somebody in the front row. I need it, too.

This whole event is about acceptance.

Yourself. (Myself.)

Your body. (My body.)

Your journey. (My journey.)

If we're able to hug a stranger, maybe we can be ready to embrace who we are when we really need it.

Now, it's time to move. We get into it a little bit, warming up the body and the mind. With so many people crammed into this room, I remind everybody that it's not about what their neighbor is doing.

"Stay committed to *your* journey," I tell them. "Your attention span is yourself. Stand on your own two feet. Look internally and take it to the next level . . . for *you*."

And, that's where we go.

After 10 minutes, the air is getting heavy. Pores are open. Breathing gets deeper, and I can hear the huffing and puffing from the stage. People are pumping it out. The energy level is high. We're still running on adrenaline and caffeine. Nobody's gassed. Yet.

I put them through a series of lunge squats, high knees, and 1-2-3 Heismans, and then I give them the bad news: "That was just the warm-up, y'all!"

Audible groaning in the room.

TRUTHBOMB: When you feel like you can't go any further, remember, *you have a reserve.* When you feel like you gotta quit, just push it that extra millisecond longer, and you show your body who's boss.

We move into a series of planks and push-ups, just like I promised, when a woman up front lets out a loud "Ohhhhhhh-hhhhhhhhhh. . . ."

She was digging seriously deep!

I run over: "Did you just say 'ohhhhh'?"

I'm messing with her.

"I'm gonna show you 'ohhhhhh.' That was just to get you engaged!"

"This is your moment," I tell her.

Tell everybody.

Tell *myself.*

"Are you going to give up, or are you going to push? Are you going to stay in? You go through this so the next time, you *know* you can make it."

Pretty soon, everybody is on their feet for switch kick punchs—fists and feet flying. Then, we go in for a few rounds of uppercuts. There's a lot of punching in my workouts, as much for the arm-and-ab workout as for the idea of it. We're all in this for the fight.

Lay a glove on that person who's got nothing but bad energy.

Put a metaphorical fist in the face of everybody holding us back, telling us "you can't," reminding us of our weaknesses.

Sure, we all have weaknesses. (I'm lookin' at *you*, M&Ms.) But, this is about finding our inner strength. And so, we keep punching until our arms are about to drop off.

TRUTHBOMB: If we can push ourselves when we're feeling weak, that's when the real progress begins.

As we jump and punch, I notice that the floor is shaking under our feet. These people are powerful.

I wonder: Are hotels in Indiana earthquake-proof?

FINALLY, THE SWEATSTORM ENDS.

What began as a sprint turned into a struggle. But, I couldn't care less if people match me move for move, or if they can only make it through 30 percent of the workout. What's important is how hard they push themselves, and how they feel right now, in the moments afterward.

At least a third are dead on their feet and hate me right now. But, I know that they don't really mean it, judging from the thanks and encouragement that are flying around the room. We've been down together, and now we're on our way back up.

At these events, we exhaust our muscles first, and then we strengthen *our minds.*

I'm channeling my Pop-Pop with his bullhorn on the streets of Camden. Preacher gonna *preach!*

"Some of you may have noticed a scar I have on my abdomen."

I flash the 3-inch scar under my belly button. People hoot.

"I got this scar when my appendix exploded, when I was working as a dancer in L.A. I couldn't eat for 2 weeks while they were figuring it out. I lost a lot of weight, and not in a good way. But, I'm telling you: Even when I weighed 175, *this didn't go away.*"

I grab a roll of flesh, covered in stretch marks, that, like my scar, I'll carry until the day I die.

"Listen, you may be on a weight-loss journey, looking to lose 10 pounds, or 20, or 40 or 60 pounds. But it's not about that number. It's not even about the weight. It's about where you'll *feel the best.* Where you can love your body. Not everybody is going to be skinny. Not everybody *should* be skinny.

"Here's where we all want to be—in a place where we feel

great. That's where you're going to look your best, because it's the best *you* there is. You don't need anything other than that, and it's impossible to have anything else, anyway. So, forget about some number on a scale. Here's the question I want you to ask yourself, because it's the same one I ask myself: How do I feel today? If the answer is 'great,' do everything you can to stay there. But, even if it's not 'great,' you still have to love yourself, just as you are today. And you have to take action toward greatness.

"You have to give if you expect to get," I continue. "Just don't expect to get much from outside yourself, because that's not where the really important stuff is coming from. Here's the key: You have to give the gifts to yourself. No one can breathe for you, right? No one can walk for you, right? No one can do a push-up for you, right?

"You're gonna do it for yourself. It's all about you being *self-ish*. I don't care if you're a mom, or you work in an office, or if you're the president of the United States. You need to focus on yourself first, help yourself first, if you want to help anybody else out."

Change of gears.

"We've just had a workout. You tired?"

Yup, they tired.

"Well, I'm tired, too. But, this isn't about whether I can do a diamond jump. And, it's not about how many of them *you* can do, either. It's not about your abs, your booty, or your biceps. It doesn't matter to me if you lost 40 pounds doing my workouts, or 5 pounds, or if you actually gained weight because you ate more while you were doing it.

"Fit comes in so many different sizes. When we think about weight, it immediately becomes a barrier. What's most important is the baggage you carry in your life. If you constantly make excuses based on your baggage, the weight is going to pour on. 'I can't do this, I can't do that *because. . . .*'

There's 5 pounds. 'Well *you* look great, but I can't do it *because.* . . .' There's 15 more pounds. Accept who you are. Where you are is where you want to be. Trust and believe in yourself . . . *right now.*

"You don't want to be saying 'I will do this,' 'I'm hoping to try that.' Say, *I can* and *I am.* You have the power right now. Live in that, breathe in that, stay in that, and don't let anyone get in your way."

If my Pop-Pop were still around, I'm pretty sure he'd give me an "Amen!"

AND NOW IT'S TIME for my favorite part of the day. The Q&A. Lots of people with their hands in the air, looking for the kind of help you don't get from a workout alone.

Do you ever get into a funk?

"Sure I do. I ask myself: Why am I in a funk? Is it external or internal? Then, I focus on the person or project I'm in a funk over. You need to be the 'antibiotic' for your own life. Attack the invader!"

How do you handle personal or emotional pain?

"There are two ways you can go: You can let it fester, or you can step out of it and go through the struggle. You gotta cry. Go across the bridge of emotion. It's terrible to go through. You didn't ask for that pain. But, you leave your mark to show your progress across that bridge. You made it to that point, and now you can move on. When you struggle, you do the work, and you get the reward. If you don't have any struggles, it's time to get out of the daisy field."

A woman takes the microphone and thanks me for helping her through a 90-pound weight loss. We all cheer for her, but she's not having any of it. She's in pain, and I can see it.

"I still check the scale every day, and I hate it when I go up a few pounds. Will this ever stop?"

"Where is your 'now'?" I ask her. "You need to accept where you are right now. You're already at your destination, and you need to be happy with that. The person you were when you weighed 90 pounds more was amazing, because she's the one who started your journey. Love that person. Go to who you are right now!"

I pick my way through the crowd, and wrap my arms around her. She needs a hug. I only wish I could time travel and hug her +90-pound self, because she's my hero. I hope she'll come to feel the same way.

Can you wrap your arms around yourself that way? You deserve that hug, that acceptance, more than you can know.

T IS FOR TRANSFORMATION

SUPERPOWER #6: FEELIN' IT

Passion is your personal mojo. If you're truly feelin' it, nothing seems impossible. If you're *not* feelin' it, nothing is possible. Passion either makes or breaks your intensity and determination. To make any new plan work, and to overcome the problems that always come when you change things up, you have to have major drive. But, too much mojo might make you bullheaded or obsessed or make you slam right into a wall. The key is to maximize the passion, minimize the crazy.

SELF-TEST: ARE YOU FEELIN' IT?

[1 = That's me! 6 = That's totally not me!]

1. Sun's up, I'm up!

1	2	3	4	5	6

2. I have a hard time relaxing and doing nothing.

1	2	3	4	5	6

3. I push myself to the max (YES!).

1	2	3	4	5	6

4. I'm restless and full of energy.

1	2	3	4	5	6

5. I'm a vigorous and passionate person.

1	2	3	4	5	6

SCORE BOX

Mostly 1s and 2s: Your mojo is workin'.

Mostly 3s and 4s: You're stuck in stop-and-go traffic.

Mostly 5s and 6s: You're just stuck.

SHAUN T'S
PASSION PLAN

EXERCISE #1

Figure out what really pisses you off. If you're emotionally dead, you're on your way to physical death as well. So, make a list of four or five things that really piss you off, and see if there's a theme that connects them. You've located your beating heart. When you need a boost, use those things you hate to create a righteous anger inside of yourself. Let it levitate you out of your funk and toward a better way. Now, build an action plan—volunteer work, a career change, new exercise goal—that keeps it pounding.

EXERCISE #2

Take a risk. Nothing stupid here, people. I don't want you to hit me up on Facebook with news that you laid your life savings on a lottery number. But, if you commit serious time and resources to a goal, you'll naturally be more passionate. Being scared sh!tless will do that for you! Put something real on the line, and your passion will be real as well.

EXERCISE #3

Locate other passionate people, and hang out with them. L.A. is a town of dreamers. And a lot of them are working their asses off to make their dreams real. Those hard workers were constantly egging me on to try harder, do more, meet new people, dream bigger dreams, and live a better reality. So, are you part of a passionate crowd, or a passive one? Remember, you're the average of the five people closest to you. Make sure those five are really *alive*!

EXERCISE #4

Give in to your obsessions. You can learn a lot from stuff you go nutty about, even if they're a little ridiculous. Okay, you follow every tweet, cat-fight, and hairdo change of the Kardashians. Sometimes, you do that in the middle of the night. What's that about? Maybe it's your career as a marketing professional about to take off. If you fill in the blank with "I can't help it, I'm obsessed with _____," you've identified a passion. Now, plot the points forward from there to see if there's a career- or life-change implied by that passion.

EXERCISE #5

Practice spontaneity. A lot of us are waiting for permission to schedule that trip, go full-out turquoise with the colorist, or run out onto the dance floor and boogie. There's no one around to grant that permission but *you*. Ask yourself: Why am I holding back? If the answer is anything but

"I'm under doctor's orders," get on with it. Right now. Shaun T will hold your place in the book while you *go a little crazy*.

EXERCISE #6

Roar. I hear it all the time. People tell me that when I yell encouragement at them during a DVD workout, they yell right back at me. And, sometimes they just cuss me out, because they can't believe how demanding I am. I'm happy with it either way. We all have too much stuff bottled up inside us, and one excellent way to pop the cork is with some scream therapy. You could do it to cheer yourself on, or you could do it to release tension, or you could just be letting the universe know how pissed you are. But, you need to let it out in a way that *you* hear it, because you're your own most important cheering section. Bust an eardrum.

Are You Too Passionate?

Then come sit next to me.

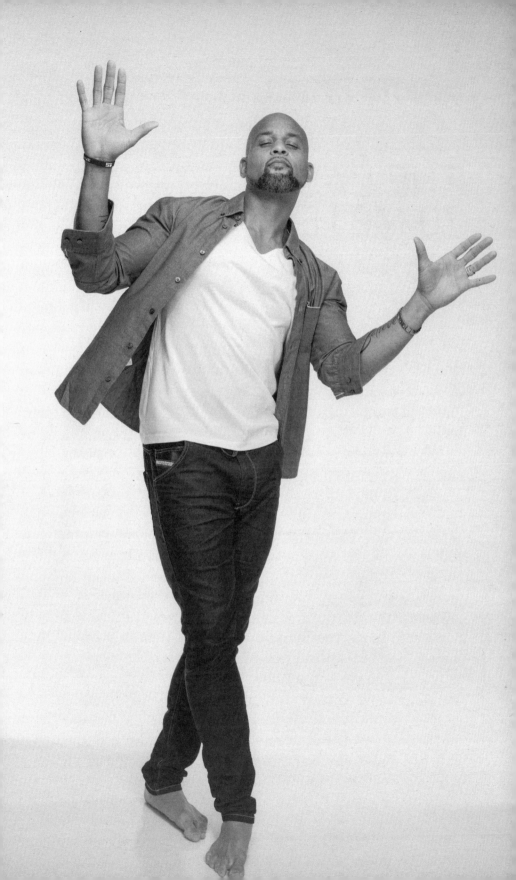

CHAPTER FIFTEEN

THE LAST 70 METERS

In track practice, we used to joke that as you rounded the final corner in the 400, one of two things would happen: You'd feel a piano drop on to your back, or rigor mortis would set in.

Which would it be? One, or both? And would we be strong enough to shrug it off and finish the last 70 meters strong?

Well that final turn is about where we are in the journey we're taking together, through this book. You've done a bunch of exercises, built (or sharpened) your tools, and I hope you're feeling good about where you are right now and where you're going.

But even as you head for the finish line, there's still a chance for the piano to crash down, or for rigor mortis to lock down your stride. They're as much a part of some races as the finish line and the cheering crowds. And most often those heavy weights come straight out of your past—the baggage you still haven't emptied; the burdens you still haven't lifted.

If you haven't, it's time—now.

The only way to guarantee your future is to deal with the past, move beyond it, and then use what you learn to help navigate your path forward.

That's how you develop the skills and tools that can help you deal with anything that comes up.

TRUTHBOMB: Because change is constant, challenges are constant, too.

The longer we live, the more tools we should accumulate, and the sharper they should become as we learn how to use them.

But only if we're doing it right.

That doesn't mean that the past is going to behave itself and stay in the past. Sometimes, it worms its way—or even explodes—back into your present, and tries to pull you backward.

Life will test you, to make sure that you've fully processed your past, that you've fully developed your superpowers, and that you're fully ready to use those tools and move on.

I've had some crazy "piano" moments that way. Because I lead a fairly public life on social media, and host public events, my personal past sometimes crashes the party. Usually, uninvited.

My biological father—remember him? The one who pushed my mom out a bathroom window?—lived on after my mother pushed him out of our lives. Flash forward to a few years ago when his sister's kid saw my *Hip Hop Abs* infomercial on TV.

This kid kept on talking to the screen—"Hi, Uncle Ennis. It's Uncle Ennis!"—and his mom kept on telling him "No, your Uncle Ennis isn't on the television."

But, finally, she took a look at the screen, and yes, there *was* a resemblance between the *Abs* guy and her brother Ennis, the man my brother was named after. And, because that guy on the screen was called Shaun T, and Ennis's last name was Thompson, she put T and T together. She reached out in her family and asked a question I guess I should have known was coming one day. "Hey, didn't Ennis have a son named Shaun back in Philly?"

Word about Shaun T finally filtered all the way down to my biological father. Given what I do for a living, I wasn't too hard to track down.

So, this guy pops up on my Facebook wall, and he looks kind of familiar. "Oh, my God!" he spouted on my wall, "You got your body from me!" He sent a picture of his six pack to my mother, who then forwarded it to me. He was 52. Okay, and fit. Congratulations. I shut that down real quick. If he didn't have time for me and my mom when I was born, I didn't have time for him now.

You can tell a lot about people by when they choose to show up. Is it just for the party, or do they pitch in with the prep work before and the clean-up afterward? Do they boost you toward success when you're starting out, or gather around to deliver "I told you sos" after something goes sideways? Do they lend a hand, or ask for a handout? One of the most difficult types of history to deal with is the flesh-and-blood kind. Just remember: who you spent time with is a choice, too.

My biological father was strictly a come-and-go guy (that is, he came, and then he went), wasn't any kind of husband to my mom, and he certainly didn't deserve the respectable title of "father." And, when he ran off the track, he passed the loser baton to a man who was even worse.

And, yes, even the stepmonster showed up again in my life, too.

Like I said, your past has a way of doing that, like in the final scene of the movie *Carrie*, when her arm thrusts up from the grave. Deal with your past, bury it deep, and plant flowers. Or, it'll pop up again and again.

I was scheduled for an event in Orlando, and he caught on to the preshow publicity, so he reached out. I got a note saying, "I hear you're going to be in town. I'd love to see you again."

What universe was he living in that he thought that was even possible?

I circulated his picture to the security guys at the event with instructions to keep him out. He didn't show up. Remember: You've got "security," too: your determination to keep your Core Five positive and supportive. Draw them close!

To this day, my only lasting regret about what happened to me from age 8 to 12 was that I didn't call out my abuser for what he did to me. If I had, I might have prevented another child from suffering as I did. Frequently, the mentality of an abuser, after a target withdraws, is "next victim." I don't know what happened when he was done with me, but I wish I had cut the chain right there.

I heard from the man who molested me one more time, near the end of his life. A relative of his passed a message that he wanted to talk to me. Maybe he had wanted to apologize to me on his deathbed? I didn't respond. That kind of confession and apology would have been more about his pain, about clearing his own conscience. Nothing he could ever say would make it up to me. The peace he sought wasn't mine to give.

When I heard that he had died, I felt exactly *nothing*. I was blank.

Now, I'm the kind of guy who, if I hit a squirrel with my car, I'm a mess for the afternoon. Tears, guilt, self-blame, grieving. But the passing of my molester was just a shadow gone from the Earth.

I had moved on, and I'm so thankful that I was able to.

It's tricky with our parents, right?

They give us life, and if they're like my mom, and like Mom-Mom and Pop-Pop, they can instill an attitude toward life and toward people that opens up the world for you. But, a parent can take away confidence, independence, and, in extreme cases, even the belief that you deserve to be loved. If your parents were missing, or they were present but toxic, it's one of the most difficult legacies to move beyond, because our parents control the soundtrack for at least our first dozen years.

All the more reason to listen carefully to the tracks they

were laying down, and decide if that's the kind of music you want to dance to for the rest of your life. If not, you owe yourself a chance to write some new music, and dance your own dance.

I'd like to compare and contrast my biological father and my abuser with my grandfather. They don't even belong in the same sentence—or on the same planet—with Pop-Pop. The Reverend Charles Dawson did so much to repair the damage from the destructive male figures in my life. As absent and negative as they were, he was that present and positive. Standing by Pop-Pop's side on the streets of Camden, listening to him preach hope, and helping him to distribute bread, he turned my eyes away from the very worst in the world and toward the very best.

I'm still looking in that direction today.

Pop-Pop passed away when I was in my early twenties. I couldn't imagine a world without Pop-Pop. But, of course, he helped me create my own world in his image.

And, in a funny way, he also helped me come to terms with who I really was back then, even though we never actually talked it through.

You remember how Pop-Pop challenged my college boyfriend, telling him that he wanted to talk to him about his "relationship" with Shaun?

We never went there in his lifetime, mostly because Mom-Mom wouldn't let that conversation happen. But, I give Pop-Pop credit for forcing *me* to think about my relationship with my first boyfriend, both to ask if this guy was right for me, but also, for pushing me to come out to my mother, to Ennis, to the rest of my world, to *myself*.

Pop-Pop might have freaked over his gay grandson; I'll never know. But, I do know that he supported me at the most vulnerable time in my life, that he and Mom-Mom taught me to trust the world again, and that he made me feel loved every day of his life.

I'm still benefiting from the gift that they gave me. They

were the strongest evidence I had that the Golden Rule could transform lives.

So, I ask you: Which parts of your past are *you* going to allow to go forward? What negatives visit you in the night, and make you question yourself? What are the positives you want to reinforce, that give you strength to meet today's load of challenges? Whose past helps you define your future in better terms? Are you strong enough to lift the piano off your back, and shake off the rigor mortis?

Are you going to reach into toxic memories, and let the people who inflicted those events on you to do their worst to you again? Or, are you going to reach into your strengths, and triumph over today's challenges with the strengths you've built over the course of your lifetime?

TRUTHBOMB: No matter how people act toward you, you alone have the power to *react.* That controls your story.

Sometimes, I laugh at people I get tangled up with in business negotiations. They try to lay things on me, try to sneak an advantage, try to intimidate me into signing an agreement or giving up my rights. I'll say to them: "Seriously? You think that stuff is going to work on me? Do you know what I've been through in my life? You're not scaring me into nothing I don't want to do!"

Then I put the sledgehammer back in my toolbox.

I know that you have one handy, too, Don't be afraid to use it when you have to.

Of course, I didn't just wake up one day and say: Now I'm done worrying about that sexual abuse. It took me years of hard work, including about 5 years of work with two therapists, to get past the guilt and the shame of it.

Usually, in the context of a workout, I'll say: Don't run from the work. *Feel* the work. Actually, that is probably even more true as you're sorting through a lifetime of slights and wounds, especially ones that happened to you when you were at your most vulnerable.

TRUTHBOMB: The more powerful the hurt you endured, the more powerful you will be when you overcome it.

Everything that happens to you—negative, positive, scary, reassuring—becomes part of the core of who you are. It can weaken you, or it can help you triumph. Over anything, or any*one*.

I STILL HAD A LOT OF stuff to sort through when I met Scott in 2010. It's one of the reasons that this book didn't come out any earlier, in fact. I hadn't written one yet, because I was telling myself: "You're so confused, and you're going to try to tell people how to lead their lives? Why should they listen to *you*?"

A workout, I could lead. Life transformation? I had a ways to go with my own transformation, first.

Here's the kind of thing I'm talking about.

Not long after I met Scott, I knew I'd be with him for the rest of my life. But, that doesn't mean it was easy for us. Far from it, and that was mostly my fault.

I'd often wake up in the middle of the night, and I'd pick a fight with him, asking if we were really meant to be together, if he really loved me.

I would say hurtful things. "This is over. This is not real." I'd challenge Scott to prove that the opposite was true.

In return, he was so kind to me.

His patience with this pattern of fights gave me time to

sort through it. So, why *was* I at my most vulnerable at the darkest time of the night?

Maybe you have a guess, but I didn't. That's another benefit of working with a therapist. They can see the patterns that you're hiding from yourself.

In one of our sessions, my therapist pointed out that my fights with Scott, as an adult, were synchronized on the clock with my abuser's drunken visits to my bedroom, when I was a child.

If that's just a coincidence, it's a mind-blowing one. And, a very sad one. Two o'clock in the morning was my personal witching hour, and I still woke up in terror, and still felt the same things that I had when I was 8 years old. It shows how persistent the past can be, messing with you for as long as you avoid it or try to push it aside.

Up until very recently, I wasn't sure I deserved somebody like Scott. Even though I had overcome so much, and succeeded beyond my wildest dreams, I wasn't sure that I deserved to be loved. I was trying to give Scott an excuse to go, to drive him off. But, he stuck with me and convinced me that I deserved him. As we did that work together, the molestation released its hold on me.

I had a present and a partner that I deserved. My sincerest wish for you is that you'll find *your* Scott.

If you're looking for a happy ending to this story, that's mine.

We'll work on yours some more in the next chapter.

What's next for me?

Still waiting for the call from Janet Jackson to go on tour.

Until then, I wake up every day looking for a way to find new challenges, be creative, and meet new people.

One of the new people I'm looking forward to meeting: Our kids, if Scott and I are lucky enough to have some. (We're trying. It's complicated. Isn't it always, if you don't have a womb handy, within the couple?)

I said that I actually enjoy a workout only when I'm completely exhausted. I hope that's when I'll really enjoy being a father, too, because I'm sure that there will be plenty of exhaustion to go around.

If we should be so fortunate. The road to starting our own family has been extremely tough. More bumps and roadblocks than we have ever encountered before. We're grateful to everybody who has pitched in so far, but there have been more downs than ups.

So, we keep on trying, keep rooting for the surrogate moms, and keep on hoping.

Of course, there are no guarantees that it'll happen for us.

Isn't that the way it goes?

Each new life phase comes with its own set of struggles. But struggle is our friend, because it's our very best motivator, and teacher, and the source of all our strength.

Bring it.

T IS FOR TRANSFORMATION

SUPERPOWER #7: BANANAS

Change and uncertainty go together like *INSANITY* and sweat. No matter how carefully you plan your life, there is always a bit of chaos. Change is not only uncomfortable, sometimes it's bananas. But that's also my favorite fruit. It's a metaphor for the craziness of life, and it comes in bunches. You can, of course, have too much "bananas," and that can make it diffi-cult to finish tasks and make decisions. But, you can learn to make bananas work for you, too.

SELF-TEST:
HOW MANY BANANAS ARE IN YOUR BUNCH?

[1 = That's me! 6 = That's totally not me!]

1. If there aren't clear answers, I'm outta here.

| 1 | 2 | 3 | 4 | 5 | 6 |

2. I'm frustrated when I can't get a grip.

| 1 | 2 | 3 | 4 | 5 | 6 |

3. When the windshield is foggy, I stop driving.

| 1 | 2 | 3 | 4 | 5 | 6 |

4. I can't stand to leave things unfinished.

| 1 | 2 | 3 | 4 | 5 | 6 |

5. I dislike vague expectations and goals.

| 1 | 2 | 3 | 4 | 5 | 6 |

SCORE BOX

Mostly 1s and 2s: You hate feeling out of control.

Mostly 3s and 4s: You like to contain the chaos.

Mostly 5s and 6s: BANANARAMA!

SHAUN T'S
BANANAS WORKOUT

EXERCISE #1

Learn about stuff. If you're uncomfortable with bananas, then peel them. Learn exactly what is going on beneath the surface. Break your crazy situation down into the individual elements, and understand every component of your unsettled situation. Reach out to others who have been where you are, taking notes and filling file folders, as necessary. Chaos can be exhilarating, in fact, if you take that feeling as encouragement to understand the chaos, and resolve it.

EXERCISE #2

Concentrate on what you *can* control. Even after you've fully explored your situation, you might still face a lot of uncertainty. It's not unusual. But, the more you work through the chaos, the more aspects of it that are actually within your control. While I was trying to launch my dance career in L.A. (a bananas enterprise if ever there was one), I stuck to what I knew in my "downtime": teaching exercise classes. The best thing about that is that it kept me fit, so when my dance career took off, I had the body to make it work. See the plan there? Decide which risks are worth taking, and prepare for them before you take the plunge. And you can just dip a toe, and then your foot and ankle, before you make the big splash.

EXERCISE #3

Exercise. Of *course,* I would tell you to work out more, right? To a guy with a hammer, everything looks like a nail. To the guy who invented *INSANITY*, everything looks like a crazy-good reason to work out. But, there's a ton of research that shows that the best answers to anxiety and depression are sweat and muscle. To help you clear your mind of chaos—I propose a bout of high-intensity interval training, often referred to by the initials HIIT. It's a mix of hard-core cardio followed by active recovery, and it is a proven calorie-burner and mental challenge. It's the foundation of many of my workouts, but you can do it without putting on one of my DVDs. If you're a runner, hit the road and sprint for 30 seconds, and follow it up with a slow jog for 2 minutes. Fifteen minutes of that will be enough for a beginner; more experienced runners can shoot for a half-hour. It'll clear your mind and give you strength and energy to turn your bananas into a fruit salad.

   Just dance. Here's why I prescribe a dance break for somebody whose life is a little out of control: When you're learning dance moves and lost in rhythm, your brain doesn't have the capacity to think about anything but the move you're doing, and the one you're about to throw yourself into. It fully occupies your attention, which can short-circuit obsessive focus on problems or worries about the outcome of a tough situation you have in play. It amazes me how often I can take a dance break and return to find that a) my problems don't seem so big when I'm done, or b) a new solution occurs to me in the shower afterward. Here are four dance moves to get you started (Turn to the appendix for detailed instructions.)

The Trip

Slide Up Down

Throw/Hands in the Air

Criss Cross

Do each move for eight 8-counts, then four 8-counts, then two 8-counts, to make a mini dance that will help you forget your worries on the way to solving them.

EXERCISE #4

Learn to live with bananas. When I set out on a new part of my own journey, it's not because I already know where I'm going to end up. It's because I *don't* know. That's where the bananas come in, but it's also where the motivation comes in: Have I prepared well enough? Am I working hard enough? Am I meeting new people? Am I learning new things? If I can honestly answer yes to all of those questions, it doesn't mean that I'll avoid the bananas that I have coming (remember, I *like* bananas), but it does guarantee that I'll end up someplace interesting and different from where I was before. And, you know what? That's the real destination. It might even be more exciting than the one you originally had in mind. That's when you'll harvest the bananas and discover just how sweet they can be.

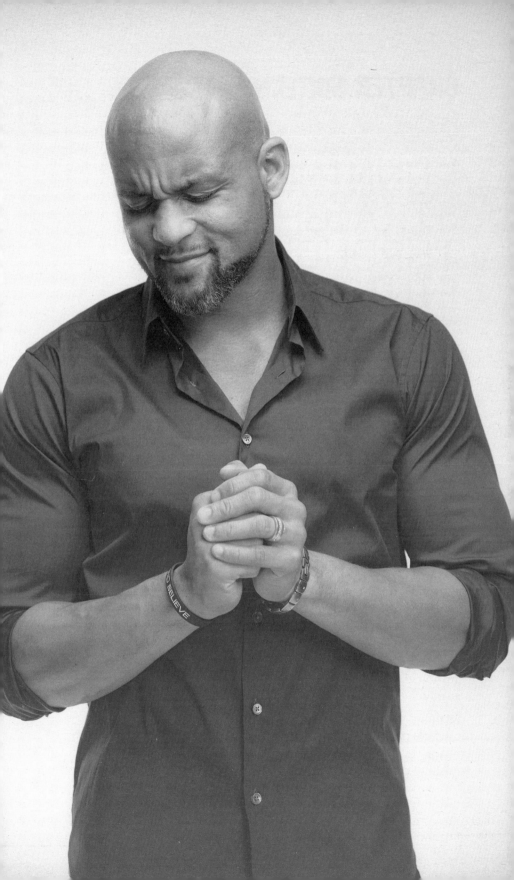

CHAPTER SIXTEEN

RUNNING STRAIGHT THROUGH THE FINISH LINE

You're headed for the end of the race.

Where are your eyes? On the tape? Or, on the track ahead?

Coach Anderson answered that one.

TRUTHBOMB: You win only if you learn to run *past* the finish line.

That may be his ultimate truthbomb.

"If you and I are running next to one another, and you stop at the tape," he told us, "I'll beat you every time. The finish line is never the finish line. If I continue my momentum and push *past* the end, I'll win because of it."

Life transformation isn't for a few months, it's a devotion you pick up now and apply to everything that happens to you until your last breath. And, that's the good news, because the more challenges you face, the more skills you'll gather, and the better every day will be from here on out.

It's not that life will become easy. You'll still have difficulties, and you'll still need to conquer them. But by cleaning up the messes as you encounter them, and sticking them permanently in your rearview mirror, you'll be able to make your present into a place you love living in.

So, it's not about the finish line, it's about the way you stride through the tape and keep on running. One finish line is replaced by another up ahead, and the run continues.

When people flash me that "after" photo, I always ask them the same question: "How does it feel?"

A lot of time, they say "great!"

But, is it really?

Only if that "after" photo is the product of an effort that you can sustain for the rest (and the best) of your life. Have you reached a place that makes you feel so good, and so comfortable with yourself, that you want to live there for the rest of your life? It doesn't mean that your work is over, but it does mean that you've found your best place, and aim to stay there.

I'm so inspired when I see people surge forward and continue their momentum into their new lives. As I've said before in this book, fit doesn't have a size, it has a mentality. That *feeling* is your goal, not any particular milestone. You want to *live your life change*, not reach some random point or achievement and stop running.

I want you to define your "beyond," and keep pumping until you run into a world that you create for yourself. Coach Anderson and I will be there to high five you at the finish line, which is also your next starting line.

Pass the baton. The new *you* will receive it, and use the momentum to move forward, always forward.

LET'S TALK ABOUT TRANSFORMATION.

You bought this book because you wanted to work on yours, and I know you can make it happen.

TRUTHBOMB: Either you accept your life as it is, or you accept your responsibility to change it.

But the person who helped you start your journey toward transformation is the strongest person you'll ever know. That's where your power comes from, and it makes you stronger than anything you need to overcome.

If you use the tools you've earned, and sharpen your skills through frequent use, you'll reach one new place, and then another, and you'll find new joys, new experiences, new people, and new belief in yourself. *You will transform yourself* into the best version of you there can be.

THE FIRST WEEKS AFTER *INSANITY* CAME out, a lot of people crashed and burned with the fit test.

"This is too hard," some people said. "I'm not doing this program."

Maybe you feel that way, and I get it. I do.

But, like the exercises and self-tests in this book, it was meant to be hard. That also means that the results you can get will be awesome. If you stick with the training, and heed your coaches, you'll make the great leap forward. Success isn't easy or quick, but it comes if you keep striving for it.

It's just what I had in mind when I created that *INSANITY* fit test, in fact. It sets a benchmark for your abilities, so you can test yourself again when you get a little farther into the program. Same with the chapter tests and exercises in this book. People are always amazed at how their capabilities improve the harder they push themselves. What was impossible today becomes achievable tomorrow, once you put in the work.

> **TRUTHBOMB:** The stronger you get, the better you feel. The better you feel, the stronger you get.

And, repeat.

Just as the *INSANITY* fit test pushed boundaries, so do the Transformation self-tests. But boundaries are there for you to cross over.

Trust and believe that you can, and you will.

Most of the work that I'm asking you to do will happen in your head, of course. That's where we build and maintain all of the barriers in our lives. But, that's also where we tear them down, and step over them.

It's your fit test for life, and, of course it's hard.

Everything worth doing takes time.

Everything worth doing is difficult.

> **TRUTHBOMB:** If your body says "quit," but your brain says "go," you *will* go, every time.

You won't quit; you will commit.

When the route is difficult but you still find a way to continue, you're also primed for progress. Vulnerability is the doorway that you pass through on your way to the life that you're meant to lead.

THAT BRINGS ME TO THE MOST important question in this book.

Why do you *need* a transformation?

Notice that I didn't say why do you *want* a transformation? Anybody could come up with a wish list that includes a 27-inch waist and a $100,000 raise. But, you probably don't need those things, it would simply be nice to have them.

What you *need* is a very different thing. It cuts to the core of who you are. You need what's essential, like food, water, shelter, and love. If you can't get what you need, you won't be able to survive. And, if your need goes that deep, nothing and nobody will be able to stand in your way as you strive to get it.

That's when transformation happens.

Often, I'll hear from somebody after a tough workout, "Thank you, Shaun T. I couldn't have gotten through that without you."

I'm happy to motivate people. That's my life's work.

But, I'm even happier when I hear somebody say, *"I found my own power."*

And then, off they go, running past the finish line to a life they couldn't quite believe was real until they made it so.

You've heard of a vicious cycle, where one bad thing leads to another and another? Well, right now you are entering into a virtuous cycle, where one strength leads to more strength, one amazeballs feeling leads to another, and you can leave Shaun T behind, because you have the power within *yourself.*

I KNOW I'M NOT THE ONLY one who has survived something terrible as a child.

My journey from abuse to redemption has been repeated many thousands of times, and because my purpose in life is to help transformations happen, I hear those kinds of stories all the time. It's my favorite part of what I do.

Every time, the answer to despair is hard work, inspiration, and finally, transformation.

To do that, you'll need to focus 100 percent on yourself. Who are you? What do you believe in? Where does your strength come from? Answer those questions and you'll identify the source of your personal power. Then no one can stop you.

Transformation begins with a mental shift—your determination to fight back.

Then, it takes on a physical component. You wake up early for a workout, or schedule a night class.

It extends into a new circle of friends and supporters who wish you the best and urge you onward.

One success comes, and then another.

And, as you feel the joy of that, you hunger for more success and employ your new skills to achieve it.

Bit by bit, small win by small win, your life is transformed, and you look around, astonished to see how far you've run past that finish line you set way back when.

At a *Shaun T Live* event, sometimes, people will tell me through tears: "You turned my life around."

And, I shed a few, too, and tell them, no, they're wrong: *"You turned your own life around."*

It all starts with **trust**, which comes from consistent action over time.

You can do that, once you know who you are and where you've come from. And, suddenly, you know where you're trying to go.

Then, when consistent action leads to progress in the direction that you've chosen, you begin to **believe**.

Now, you're locked on the path forward and upward.

I'm more certain of your success than I am that $2 + 2 = 4$.

Trust.

And believe.

You can achieve anything you set your mind to.

I know you can do this.

It's transformation time.

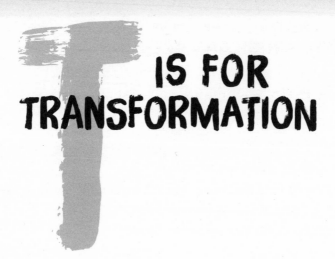

IS FOR TRANSFORMATION

THE ULTIMATE "T IS FOR TRANSFORMATION" TEST: DO YOU TRUST AND BELIEVE?

When you trust and believe, you have faith in yourself right now, and you look upward toward a better future. That immediately puts you in the circle of people who are looking in the same direction, and your energy and belief feeds off theirs. You're in a max-out multiplier, and trust and belief grow even more.

Now, nothing can stop you.

So now it's time to trust and believe.

SELF-TEST:
DO YOU TRUST AND BELIEVE?

[1 = That's me! 6 = That's totally not me!]

1. When something good happens to somebody else, I think of reasons that they don't deserve it.

1	2	3	4	5	6

2. When I hear good news, I brace myself for the disaster that always follows.

1	2	3	4	5	6

3. Hope is just a small town in Arkansas.

1	2	3	4	5	6

4. Unless I am guaranteed success for my move, I stay put.

1	2	3	4	5	6

5. If somebody does me a favor, I wonder what they're really after.

1	2	3	4	5	6

SCORE BOX

Mostly 1s and 2s: Outlook doubtful

Mostly 3s and 4s: Keep hope alive!

Mostly 5s and 6s: True believer

SHAUN T'S
TRUST-AND-BELIEVE
REGENERATION PLAN

EXERCISE #1

Learn to forgive (yourself and others). You ever see a sprinter in the Olympics, towing his suitcase down the track? Does Serena Williams step up to the service line with her tennis bag around her neck? Does Superman fly with carry-on baggage? No, no, and no. So, why are you carrying around all those heavy resentments and regrets? People have harmed you, thwarted you, insulted you. It happens to all of us. But, if you try to move forward, while still looking back at the people who did you wrong, you're going to run into wall after wall. Likewise, if you're spending precious effort keeping a list of your own failures, you're wasting energy that you could be putting toward your next success. Don't give the power to the people who did you wrong, or feel diminished by the ways you didn't measure up. Instead, forgive the trespassers, forget the times you messed up, and *move on*. You'll be amazed at how light a step you have as you sprint forward.

EXERCISE #2

Put trust to the test. There's only one way to build more trust into your life, and that's to be a more trusting person. I'm not telling you to hand out your ATM password to strangers. I'm suggesting that you practice, in small ways at first, putting more faith in the people around you. Find a friend to do a physical challenge with, like training for a 10-K or joining a boot camp or signing up for a 12-week course together. Make yourself vulnerable by letting that person see you struggle. Sure, you may get burned a few times as you expand your circle of trust. Keep at it anyway. The only way to teach trustworthiness is to practice trust, and the more trust you put out in your world, the bigger the circle of trust you'll build. And, when you trust yourself, and have a posse of people who trust you and who you can trust, you have everything you need to build the world you've dreamed of.

EXERCISE #3

Show your true colors. Stop covering things up because you don't think the world can accept them. A bad aspect of your past. The debt you're struggling to repay. A toxic relationship with a parent, sibling, or spouse. A dream that you're afraid others will make fun of. An eating problem you deny. Shame about your body. Whatever it might be, if you're covering it up, you're giving it power over you. So, dig up what you've buried, and find a way to accept it. Find a way to accept yourself. And then be honest with the world. You don't need to go full Kardashian here and overshare on Facebook, but you do need to be real with the people who matter most to you. And, if they can't love the real you, find people who can. They're out there, and being honest with yourself and others is the only way to find them, and live fully as *you*.

EXERCISE #4

Give judgment a rest. The world is a complicated place. Your own personal history is probably filled with complications. All of that can motivate a lot of different actions in life. We can leap to conclusions about those actions—by ourselves, by others—without fully understanding them. So, give the temptation to judge, to blame, a rest. Forgive the trespasses—your own, and others. If you don't judge yourself or others, you can purge so much poison from your life. Move on. You just dropped the heaviest burden you carry. Now, you can go anywhere.

EXERCISE #5

Show up on time. It seems like a small thing, right? When you say that you'll meet a friend for lunch at noon, arrive at 11:55. When you tell your kid you'll go to the park on Saturday morning, make the picnic sandwiches the night before. When you tell your boss that the report will be on her desk on Tuesday afternoon, deliver it at noon. Your personal commitments are a big deal. They tell people how much you value them. And, when you honor commitments, you build the amount of trust in your world. If people believe that you're good for the small stuff, they know you can be trusted for the big stuff, too. And, that's what all of these "Trust and Believe" exercises are about: Building the amount of trust in your world. Set an example by being trust*worthy*, and watch people reflect that back at you. Even when they don't, you'll know that *you're* behaving the right way, and so you'll come to trust yourself. That's the most important belief there is.

EXERCISE #6

Offer (and accept) help, no questions asked. People broadcast their approach to life, and their signals come through loud and clear everywhere they go. That's another way of looking at karma: The vibe you give out returns to you, only louder, because it's amplified by all the people in your life. So that's why I recommend committing yourself to some kind of volunteer work. You don't have to go into the soup kitchen, or hand out bread on the sidewalk like my Pop-Pop did, but, if you look around, you'll find plenty of opportunities to help, from distracting the crabby toddler in the grocery cart in front of you, to helping the 89-pound granny hoist her luggage into the rack above her seat on the airplane. Sure, you're busy. I am, too. But, if you put your helping hands to work in the world, you can believe that other helping hands will return the favor. In fact, one of the surest ways to make a friend is to ask a favor, and then repay it. And, offer your help as a gift. Don't expect anything back in return. It fills your world with good karma, which is a reward in itself. It's trust and belief in action.

EXERCISE #7

Let it go. This might be the most important one of all. If you want a new start, make a break with your past. Those emotional burdens that exhaust you carrying them around? Drop them, now. Loosen your grip on a grudge, become forgetful about feuds. Start over with an enemy, or just lay down your weapons and leave the battlefield. It takes a lot of energy to stay angry at someone, to replay the hurts and insults in your mind, to find new reasons to stay mad. And, the more you dwell on that stuff, the less energy you have to love and forgive yourself, and to find the people who are worth your own love and forgiveness. A long-running fight allows your enemies to take over your life, so just stop fighting. It halves your enemies' strength, and doubles yours. So, make like Queen Elsa in *Frozen*, and let it go. We all need more warmth in this big old chilly world.

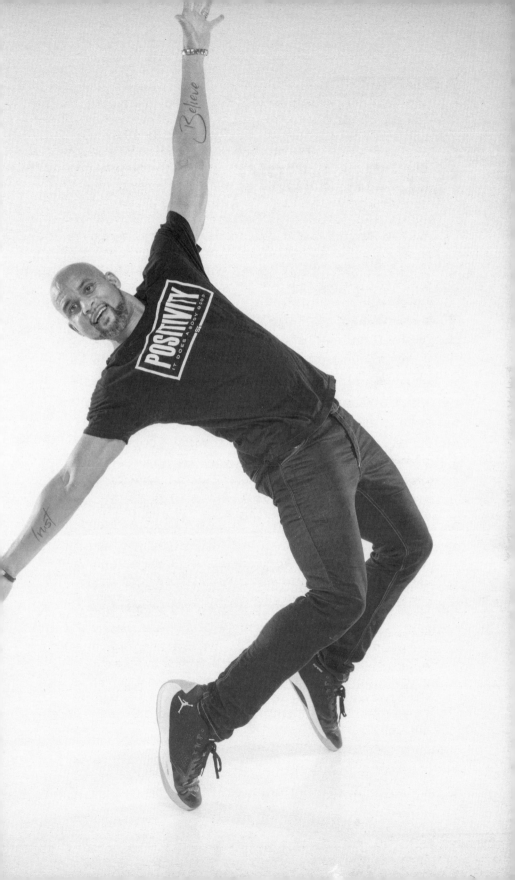

APPENDIX

FEEL THE WORK!

I've said that the most important work any of us does happens inside us—in our hearts and minds. Make progress there, and it will radiate throughout your body and your life.

But, there's a reason that I've spent my whole life as a fitness coach and motivator: Sweating through a workout can force you to dig deep, and give you the kind of change you can see. I'm still enjoying the benefits of the first 4 pounds I lost, going from 228 to 224 and feeling so good because of it.

So, here I'll share an abs plan and a body-weight cardio workout, and give you a little dance you can do to celebrate all of your progress (and burn serious calories, if you really work it).

So right here, you'll find everything you need to work on the transformation within and shine up the outside as well. The two can operate together to make a whole new you.

WORKOUT: GO NUCLEAR

How many times have you told yourself: I just don't have time for a full workout today. So, you blow it off, check your e-mail 75 times, sit in the Starbucks drive-thru, see what I'm up to on Instagram. It's okay, I get it. You're busy! But, if you happen to have just 5 minutes, you can go into a full meltdown with Shaun T's body-weight "Go Nuclear" workout. Think of the engineers and office workers I trained at the power plant in New Jersey, and touch off a chain reaction of life improvement. First, tune your mental soundtrack to 100 percent pure positivity. (Maybe turn on an actual one, if you have a favorite 5-minute song. Personally, I'd hit play on "Alive" by Krewella, "Chandelier" by Sia, "Here" by Alessia Cara, "Firestone" by Kygo, or "What Do You Mean?" by Justin Bieber.) Your muscles and lungs won't get you through this, your *mind* will.

POWER KNEES

Assume a wide stance, knees bent slightly. Shift your weight onto your right leg, lowering into a shallow squat. Kick the left leg out to the side, and lift your arms over your head. Squeeze your abs and bring your left knee toward your chest. Touch your hands to your knee at the highpoint, then return your foot to the ground. Repeat for 30 seconds, then switch sides.

POWER JACKS

Stand with your feet shoulder-width apart, back straight, arms at your sides. Hop your feet out to the sides and drop into a squat. Pressing into your heels, jump up, bring your feet together, and touch your hands over your head. Then hop back to the starting position, with your feet shoulder-width apart. Continue jacking for 60 seconds.

POWER JUMPS

Squat with your heels flat and your hands in ready position at your sides. Jump into the air, bringing your knees up, and clapping your hands against your thighs. Make a soft landing, hands back to your sides, and then repeat for 60 seconds.

POWER PUSH-UPS

Assume a high plank position, your hands under your shoulders, core tight, head in neutral position, and butt flat. Lower your body until your chest grazes the floor, then push back up. Do as many as you can for 1 minute. Almost at meltdown, now.

POWER SQUATS

Go into a shallow crouch with your toes facing forward, heels on the ground, legs hip-width apart. Your chest should be up, your back flat, and your arms at your side. Drop into a squat, swinging your arms forward as you go. Raise back up into the starting position. Continue until you reach China Syndrome, or 1 minute, whichever comes first.

WORKOUT: TIP-TOP ABS

I've always been grateful to my midsection, because core strength made me the man that I am today. It brought me back from a 50-pound weight gain, and it saved me when my appendix exploded. Seeing as I owe it all to my abs, it's my duty to give a six pack back to the world. Here are my top five exercises for core strength. No, you don't have to have abs to be fit, or show off your six pack to be sexy. But, you might want them to prevent back pain, improve your posture, or make you better at sports (okay, sex, too). Whatever your reason, I'm your abdominal answer man. Do each of these for 5 minutes a day, and it might deliver that six pack you've been waiting for. If not, no worries. Core strength is good no matter how you wear it.

SWITCH KICK PUNCH

Assume a fighter's stance with your left foot forward. Kick with your right leg and punch with your left fist. Switch legs and arms, jump kicking with your left leg and punching with your right fist. Continue alternating without returning to the starting position.

ALTERNATING TOE TAP

Assume a plank position with your feet together, arms straight, and hands positioned below but slightly wider than your shoulders. Touch your left foot to your right hand. Repeat, this time touching your right foot to your left hand. Continue alternating.

OBLIQUE KNEE TAPS

Assume a side-plank position with your weight on your left forearm, your body straight, and your right hand in front of your chest, palm facing your feet. Touch your right knee to your right hand. Return to the starting position and repeat. Switch sides each round.

PUNCHING ABS

Assume a c-sit position, with your butt and heels on the floor, knees bent, and torso at a 45-degree angle. Lift your feet 3″ off of the floor, maintaining the c-sit position. Now bring your right fist to your side and use your stomach as a punching bag, alternating left and right fists into your abs.

PIKE-UP SPIDER LUNGE

Assume a plank position and walk your feet closer to your hands so your body forms an upside-down V. Step forward with your right foot, bringing it next to your right hand, while pushing your left foot back to the running lunge position. Hop back into pike up position and hop into a running lunge, now with your left foot forward next to your left hand. Continue alternating. The rhythm for this move is—hop into pike up—hop into spider lunge (right foot forward)—hop into pike up—hop into spider lunge (left foot forward).

WORKOUT: DANCE YOUR ASS OFF

YOU SAY YOU CAN'T DANCE, but you can brush your teeth, right? Mop the kitchen floor? Haul the trash out to the curb? Well, if you can do any of those things, you can *CIZE* it up as well.

Right after my *CIZE* workout was released in 2015, I was on *Live! with Kelly and Michael* teaching them how to add a beat and dance steps to everyday activities so they're amazeballs, not boring. Polishing your molars never felt this good or burned this many calories, if you just put some movement into it! Feed something upbeat into your headphones and try Shaun T's 4-step dance meltdown. Do each move for eight 8-counts, then four 8-counts, then two 8-counts, to make a mini dance that will give you a max workout in just a few minutes.

It may feel awkward at first, but even awkward can be good exercise. Then, as you progress, throw your heart and body into it. It's the most fun you can have, while still burning a ton of calories.

MOVE #1: THE TRIP

Remember that time you tripped over a crack in the street and no one saw you? That's the inspiration for this move! Fall forward onto your left leg, bending your knee and letting your upper body rock forward, as well. Your right leg extends back in the air at the same time. Your right hand also falls forward pointing toward the ground (like you were going to catch yourself if you *really* fell). Hop onto your left leg as you swing your extended right leg in front of your body with a flexed foot, leaning back and engaging your core. Repeat this movement letting the leg kick back and forth as you "trip" onto your standing leg. Arms should move naturally with your body.

MOVE #2: SLIDE DOWN UP DOWN

Step out with your right foot (like you are moving out of the way because someone just tried to run you over!). As you step out of the way, windmill your arms up over your head. Bring your left leg together with your right and do an adductor demi-squat while closing your arms together in a genie arm position (one arm on top of the other—make a wish!). In the low genie tuck squat position, come up standing, leaving your arms crossed and popping your chest out and back while you return to the genie adductor squat position. Now it's time to go back to the left side, repeating everything you did to get to the right—step out with your left foot, windmilling your arms and going into an adductor genie squat, come up standing and pop your chest in and out as you return down to the adductor genie squat. Repeat side to side. The rhythm should feel like slide-down-up-down . . . slide-down-up-down.

MOVE #3: THE THROW/HANDS IN THE AIR

Step to the side onto your left leg, keeping on the ball of the foot and twisting your heel out. Lean back and throw your arms out like you just pushed someone really hard and said: "Get off me, bro!" Return to the center and repeat on the right-hand side (Step out, "Get off me, bro!"—right side) Do each throw one time on each side. Then, take the throw toward the sky above your head, instead of out front of your chest. Repeat on both sides. The rhythm is throw left . . . throw right . . . throw sky left . . . throw sky right. Remember to swing forcefully and lean the body back as you throw your arms in the air.

MOVE #4: CRISS CROSS

Standing with feet apart, draw your right arm across your body with a fist toward your left shoulder. Draw the left arm in toward the right shoulder making the arms cross in front of the chest. Punch the right arm down by your side. Punch the left arm down by your side. Jump and cross the feet in front of each other. Jump back out into a wide stance. Drop the head into the hands bending the body forward into a squat. Stand up. Repeat. Entire move should take 1 count of 8—for example, cross right arm across the chest (1 count), cross the left arm across the chest (1 count). . . . and so on. There you have it! LIVE IN THOSE 8s!

TiME TO PASS THE BATON . . .

YOU'VE DONE IT!

You've made it to the end.

But the good student you are knows that this is a new beginning.

Go back to the notes you took, or the chapters that spoke to you, or the Truthbombs that hit you hardest, and incorporate them into your life.

Pass the baton to the new you, waiting to sprint into your new life.

I know you can, because you reached this spot.

Trust and believe in you.

I sure do.

You can do this!

ACKNOWLEDGMENTS

Thank you, everyone. You are all so special to me . . . even if we have never met before.

INDEX